MW01415261

PRAISE FOR

DEPROGRAM DIET CULTURE

"It is with clarity and wisdom that *Deprogram Diet Culture* takes anyone struggling with dieting, food, and eating on an engaging journey of awakening. Dr. Supatra Tovar skillfully weaves together real-life anecdotes, behavioral change practices, the power of mindfulness, and cutting-edge research to give readers the tools necessary to transform their experience with food, dieting, and body. If you want to get off the diet merry-go-round and heal your relationship with food, look no further. *Deprogram Diet Culture* is a pathbreaking book for realizing the peace, balance, and joy that are inherent in each bite and morsel."

—**DONALD ALTMAN**, MA, LPC, former vice president, The Center for Mindful Eating; best-selling author, *The Mindfulness Toolbox, Simply Mindful, Meal by Meal,* and *Simply Mindful Resilience*

"In the fitness world, we often grapple with the perplexing maze of diets, each promising miracles but leaving us in a tizzy of guilt and shame. Dr. Tovar's book is a breath of fresh air, guiding you to break free from the dieting hamster wheel. It's not just about shedding pounds; it's about reshaping your relationship with food and yourself. For anyone tired of the endless cycle of dieting, this book is your ticket to a healthier, happier you, without ever having to diet again!"

—**TRACEY MALLETT**, world-renowned fitness and wellness expert; best-selling author of *Sexy in 6* and *Super Fit Mama*; creator of workouts bootybarre and bbarreless

"As a woman whose career is centered in entertainment, I know firsthand what the demands of Diet Culture have produced in the way of insecurity in what perfection is supposed to look like, and I highly recommend *Deprogram Diet Culture* as a way of reimagining our relationships to food and ourselves."

—**NOELLE SCAGGS,** co-lead singer of Fitz and The Tantrums, Scaggs Entertainment, Inc.

"Dr. Tovar shows us how to break free from unhealthy relationships with food to develop peace and power from a healthy relationship with eating. The key to the wisdom she provides is her integration of personal experiences, case examples, and the science of psychology. *Deprogram Diet Culture* is rational guidance in a world of senseless dieting."

—**DR. WILLIAM JULY,** licensed clinical psychologist, national best-selling author

"From my journey exploring cheap eats to gourmet treats, I know the pressure of maintaining health when working in the food industry. *Deprogram Diet Culture* is a lifeline, offering realistic and healthy approaches to food while never losing the fun and joy that comes with eating and enjoying every single bite."

—**ALI KHAN,** television host on Food Network, Cooking Channel, PBS, and History Channel; food writer for *The Takeout, Texas Highways,* and *Ali Khan Eats*

"After teaching cooking and healthy eating for so many years, I was surprised to learn that Dr. Supatra Tovar's book has completely opened my mind to a new way of looking and thinking about food. I instantly implemented the changes and noticed how I started to enjoy eating and had a better and healthier relationship with food. Dr. Supatra Tovar's approach is wise, compassionate, full of common sense, and easy. I recommend everyone reads this book as it will improve your relationship with food and make you feel better about yourself (and as a side effect, you will come back to your normal weight without worrying about it). A must-read!"

—ALEXANDER GERSHBERG, award-winning chef; cooking teacher; author of *Vegan for Friends, Energy,* and *Plantbased* cookbooks

"As a fellow psychologist, nutritionist, and passionate advocate for women's well-being, I'm delighted to endorse *Deprogram Diet Culture* by Dr. Supatra Tovar. This book brilliantly addresses the unique challenges women face with dieting, especially during midlife. It offers a refreshing perspective on why diets fail and guides you toward a healthier, more sustainable relationship with food and yourself. Buy this book and ditch dieting forever."

—DR. ELLEN ALBERTSON, The Midlife Whisperer®

"As a professor committed to improving individual and community health, I appreciate the approach of *Deprogram Diet Culture*. Dr. Tovar's book offers practical, science-based strategies for lifelong healthy eating habits, free from the constraints of traditional dieting."

—DR. KATHRYN HILLSTROM, EdD, MPH, RDN, FAND, professor and chair, Department of Nutrition and Food Science, California State University, Los Angeles

"As an eating disorder survivor and previous co-owner of an eating disorder clinic, I found Dr. Tovar's *Deprogram Diet Culture* extremely insightful, educational, and helpful for those struggling with their relationship with food. The practices within the book are explained in a way that makes them accessible to anyone on their journey to break free from Diet Culture. A must-read for anyone who's ready to live a life of food freedom while nourishing and honoring their body!"

—**NATALIE LEON**, wellness speaker, fitness and body image advocate

"As a trainer who values the importance of integrating science-based perspectives to educate how we create change in our body, I applaud *Deprogram Diet Culture* for incorporating this empowering approach. Dr. Tovar's book provides this valuable support and much-needed encouragement to redefine our relationship with food and self."

—**KIMBERLY SPENCER**, joint mobility and Pilates specialist

"In her kind, compassionate, and insightful style, Dr. Tovar's knowledgeable approach emphasizes mindfulness and awareness to help readers manage their physical and mental wellness healthily. Bravo!"

—**MARÍA BOTERO OMARY**, PhD, MPP, principal, The Omary Group; former faculty member, Departments of Human Nutrition and Food Science, Cal Poly Pomona and California State University Los Angeles

"In this easily digestible book, Dr. Tovar helps readers take the stress out of eating. Her focus on mindfulness and behavioral change science are invaluable for anyone wanting to stop dieting and finally start living."

—CHANTAL DONNELLY, physical therapist; best-selling author of *Settled: How to Find Calm in a Stress-Inducing World*

"Dr. Tovar's book, *Deprogram Diet Culture*, has saved me from the crushing influences of today's diet-driven culture. With easy-to-understand bites of science, psychology, and real-life stories, she has taught me that no food is bad, perfection is an illusion, and that I am worthy. The book teaches how to use small achievable steps to gain a healthier relationship with food and ultimately myself by bringing mindfulness and balance into my daily journey with food. I have learned to slow down my eating, enjoy all foods, and to not look at my body in the formerly negative fashion that has plagued me for a long time. This new way of thinking has helped me to maintain a healthy body weight and improved my self-esteem and overall compassion with the world around me. From my personal experience, I highly recommend *Deprogram Diet Culture* to anyone struggling with the pressures of our hyper-intensive diet culture as a way to break free and start a meaningful new relationship with food and yourself."

—SCOTT PEEBLES, television video editor

DEPROGRAM DIET CULTURE

Rethink Your Relationship
with Food, Heal Your Mind,
and Live a Diet-Free Life

DR. SUPATRA TOVAR
Clinical Psychologist, Registered Dietitian, and Fitness Expert

Foreword by WELDON LONG
New York Times *and* Wall Street Journal *best-selling author*

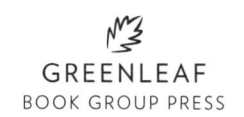

GREENLEAF
BOOK GROUP PRESS

This book is intended as a reference volume only, not as a medical manual. The information given here is designed to help you make informed decisions about your health. It is not intended as a substitute for any treatment that may have been prescribed by your doctor. If you suspect that you have a medical problem, you should seek competent medical help. You should not begin a new health regimen without first consulting a medical professional.

The names and identifying characteristics of persons referenced in this book have been changed to protect their privacy.

Deprogram Diet Culture®, ANEW Insight®, Advanced Nutrition and Emotional Wellness®, and the ANEW logo are registered trademarks of Advanced Nutrition and Emotional Wellness, LLC. Unlawful use is prohibited.

Copyright registered. All rights reserved. No part of this publication may be reproduced, distributed, or transmitted in any form or by any means, including photocopying, recording, or other mechanical or electronic methods, without the prior written permission of the publisher, except for use as brief quotations embodied in critical reviews and certain other noncommercial use as permitted by copyright law. To request permission, contact ANEW at the following address:

Advanced Nutrition and Emotional Wellness, LLC
301 N. Lake Ave, Suite 600
Pasadena, CA 91101

connect@anew-insight.com

Published by Greenleaf Book Group Press
Austin, Texas
www.gbgpress.com

Copyright © 2024 Dr. Supatra Tovar

All rights reserved.

Thank you for purchasing an authorized edition of this book and for complying with copyright law. No part of this book may be reproduced, stored in a retrieval system, or transmitted by any means, electronic, mechanical, photocopying, recording, or otherwise, without written permission from the copyright holder.

Distributed by Greenleaf Book Group

For ordering information or special discounts for bulk purchases, please contact Greenleaf Book Group at PO Box 91869, Austin, TX 78709, 512.891.6100.

Design and composition by Greenleaf Book Group and Sheila Parr
Cover design by Greenleaf Book Group and Sheila Parr
Cover images © Shutterstock/ElenaChelysheva, Shutterstock/ Christine Schmidt, and iStockphoto/seregam

Publisher's Cataloging-in-Publication data is available.

Print ISBN: 979-8-88645-194-8

eBook ISBN: 979-8-88645-195-5

To offset the number of trees consumed in the printing of our books, Greenleaf donates a portion of the proceeds from each printing to the Arbor Day Foundation. Greenleaf Book Group has replaced over 50,000 trees since 2007.

Printed in the United States of America on acid-free paper

24 25 26 27 28 29 30 31   10 9 8 7 6 5 4 3 2 1

First Edition

I dedicate this book to my loving husband, Alberto.

*Thank you for being my rock, my partner,
and my greatest supporter.
Without you, none of this would have been possible.*

I love you.

DISCLAIMER: THIS BOOK DOES NOT PROVIDE INDIVIDUALIZED HEALTH-CARE ADVICE AND DOES NOT GUARANTEE ANY OUTCOME.

The information provided herein is for informational and educational purposes only and only for your use. This material is not intended to be a substitute for professional medical advice, diagnosis, or treatment for mental health therapy provided by a licensed health-care practitioner. Always seek and obtain the advice of a qualified healthcare provider when you have questions regarding a treatment or a physical or mental condition and before undertaking a new healthcare regimen. Never disregard professional medical or psychological advice or delay seeking it because of something you have read in the materials offered by Advanced Nutrition and Emotional Wellness, LLC (ANEW). Scientific studies and research cited in this book are gathered from reputable sources. Although every reasonable precaution has been made to ensure the accuracy of the information, no guarantee can be given that the information is free from error or omission. Neither ANEW nor Dr. Supatra Tovar is responsible for any errors or omissions in reporting or explanation. No one should use the information, resources, or tools contained within these materials to self-diagnose or self-treat any health-related condition, including any eating disorder. Neither ANEW nor Dr. Tovar give any assurance, representation, or warranty regarding the accuracy, authenticity, completeness, timeliness, or applicability of the content. Not everyone can expect to have the exact same results. If you find information that is incorrect, please contact connect@anew-insight.com.

If you think you may be having a medical emergency, call your doctor or the appropriate emergency number immediately. If you are currently receiving treatment, please continue to follow the terms of your treatment until advised otherwise by your health-care provider. If you have or suspect you may have an eating disorder, please consult your health-care provider or the National Eating Disorders Association Helpline at 1-800-931-2237. If you are a minor, you should consult with your legal guardian or an adult when considering treatment and treatment providers.

CONTENTS

Foreword xiii

Acknowledgments xvii

Preface xxi

Introduction 1

Chapter 1: Stop the Diet Hamster Wheel. 5

Chapter 2: Redefining Your Ideal Food Relationship 29

Chapter 3: Hunger and Fullness vs. Emotional
or Mindless Eating 47

Chapter 4: You Are Your Own Worst Enemy—
How to Be Your Best Friend 65

Chapter 5: The Present Moment Is a Gift 85

Chapter 6: Tiny Steps for Success. 101

Chapter 7: Adding on and Preventing Relapse 119

Glossary 141

Notes 147

Index 155

About the Author 169

FOREWORD

When my dear friend Tony Capullo recently asked me to meet with a friend of his about a book she wrote on Diet Culture, I thought to myself, *What the hell do I know about diet and nutrition?*

After all, I have spent my career writing and speaking on the topics of business development and sales. I am also a 60-year-old man who has struggled with diet and weight my entire life. I grew up in the South with eating habits that were more deadly than healthy.

How the hell can I contribute to a discussion on health and nutrition—other than, perhaps, being an example of what NOT to do? Nevertheless, as a favor to my friend I agreed to meet Dr. Tovar.

She had me at "there are no bad foods!"

As the good doctor began explaining her decades-long career in nutrition, fitness, and clinical psychology and her approach to healthier living, I knew EXACTLY why my friend wanted us to speak. We were, in a way, kindred spirits.

You see, my speaking and writing career has revolved around the idea that success in business and sales is primarily a mindset issue more so than a behavioral issue. After all, our behaviors are simply reflections and neurological reactions to our thoughts, so if we want to drive behaviors that are conducive with business and financial success, we simply have to change our thoughts first.

As my dear friend the late Stephen R. Covey once said, "If you want temporary change, focus on your behaviors. If you want permanent change, focus on your thoughts."

So, after speaking with Dr. Tovar, I readily agreed to read her new book, *Deprogram Diet Culture: Rethink Your Relationship with Food, Heal Your Mind, and Live a Diet-Free Life*, more from a perspective of self-interest than as a favor to my friend Tony.

And boy am I glad I did. And you will be too.

As I read the book, I realized that my habits of mindless eating and often labeling certain foods as "the enemy" and occasionally even as "the devil" were what was really holding me back. I began to feel a profound relief. My struggle with healthy eating wasn't nearly as much a physiological struggle as it was a mindset struggle. And overcoming challenges and struggles by creating a better mindset was something I knew a great deal about. I had actually written two books on the subject.

All I had to do was to approach my behaviors and relationship with food from a perspective of changing my mindset.

And so there it was. My epiphany. The understanding that I had a mindset issue with food was liberating because I have 100 percent control over my thoughts. And with a little work around being mindful about my eating and changing my habitual thoughts around food with a simple mantra or two was a game changer.

So read this book and relax. You don't have to struggle. You can change your thoughts around food. And when you change your thoughts around food, you will change your emotions around food. And when you change your emotions around food, you will change your behaviors around food. And when you change your behaviors around food, you will change your results.

May you read this book in good health.

—Weldon Long, author of the *New York Times* and *Wall Street Journal* bestseller *The Power of Consistency* and *The Upside of Fear*

ACKNOWLEDGMENTS

In the remarkable journey of writing *Deprogram Diet Culture*, I have been graced with unwavering support that has served as my guiding star, instrumental in the completion of this book. The invaluable guidance and encouragement from several exceptional individuals have been essential to this endeavor. Without their support, the realization of this book would not have been possible.

My first thank-you goes to my husband, Alberto. The countless hours you devoted, not merely in presence, but in the immeasurable depths of understanding, wisdom, and love, have been the bedrock upon which this endeavor found its strength. Your hand, always there to hold, provided solace in moments of doubt and fatigue. Your wisdom, a beacon in times of uncertainty, illuminated the path when the complexities of this subject wove a challenging tapestry. But most importantly, your love, unending and all-embracing, became the sanctuary where my ideas and convictions found their voice. I am so grateful for the life we made and the family we created with Max, Charlie, and baby angel Huey.

Additionally, my deepest gratitude goes to my brother Robert Hanna, whose creative insight, exceptional design skills, and profound technical knowledge have been indispensable in bringing this book and course to fruition. Robert, your artistic vision and technical prowess have not only shaped the aesthetic and functional aspects of this project but have also added a layer of depth and professionalism that only your unique talents could provide. Your support, both emotionally and professionally, has been a cornerstone of this endeavor. Your involvement has transformed these projects from mere concepts into tangible realities, elevating them to a level I could not have achieved alone. Thank you, Robert, for your unwavering support and for being such an integral part of this journey. Your contributions have been nothing short of vital, and I am immensely grateful for everything you have done.

To my beloved family—my mother and father, whose unwavering support has been the bedrock of my journey, and to my sister, who has been my guide and mentor from my earliest memories, including the fundamental lesson of brushing my teeth. This book and course, significant milestones in my career, owe much to the foundational values and lessons you have instilled in me. Your endless encouragement, love, and belief in my abilities have not only shaped who I am but have also been vital in making this project a reality. Your support has been a constant source of strength and inspiration, guiding me through every challenge and celebrating every success. To you, my family, I extend my deepest gratitude and love, for you have been the guiding stars in this endeavor and in my life. Thank you for everything.

To the exceptional team at Greenleaf Book Group, my heartfelt gratitude is immeasurable. The journey of bringing my work to life has been an enriching experience, largely due to your unparalleled commitment, expertise, and passion. To

Jen Glynn, Morgan, Heather, Pam, Erin, Amanda, Danielle, Gwen, Sheila, Erin, Neil, Jen Rios, Kristine, and Justin—each of you and everyone at Greenleaf has played a vital role in this endeavor, contributing your unique talents and unwavering support. Your collective efforts have not only enhanced the quality of my work but also made this process a memorable and rewarding one. My sincerest thanks to you all for being the best publishing team one could ever hope for.

This book and course, both milestones in my professional journey, would not have been possible without the invaluable contributions of my esteemed friends and colleagues. To Chantal Donnelly, PT, whose insights in physical therapy have been foundational; Dr. Ellen Miller-Kwon, whose wisdom and expertise have guided critical aspects of this work; Deborah Rosen, whose support has been unwavering; Dash Holland Corpe, RD, whose nutritional expertise has enriched this project; Dr. Arianne Tang, whose knowledge and perspective have been instrumental; Nancy Tsai, whose collaboration has been vital; Sharon Bowers, RD, for her invaluable input on dietary matters; and Scott Peebles, whose contributions have been essential to the success of this endeavor. Your collective expertise, support, and dedication have not only made this project a reality but have also significantly enhanced its quality and impact. Thank you all for your invaluable contributions and for being a part of this journey.

A special dedication to Tony Capullo, the man with the network and the heart to connect me to Weldon Long, whose foreword graces my book. Weldon, with his transformative journey from adversity to success, embodies the very essence of changing mindsets—a core theme that resonates deeply with both our works. His belief in the power of consistency and a prosperity mindset mirrors our shared passion for fostering positive change in the lives of others.

Finally, a profound and heartfelt acknowledgment to my clients, who have been integral to this journey. Each meeting with you is not just a session, but an opportunity for mutual growth and learning. Your experiences, challenges, and triumphs have not only enriched my professional perspective but have also been a source of continuous inspiration. This book and course, crafted with the insights gained from our interactions, stand as a testament to the valuable lessons you impart. Without you, this achievement would not have been conceivable. You are not just clients; you are collaborators in the truest sense, and for this, I am eternally grateful. Thank you for being a pivotal part of this journey and for enabling the creation of work that reflects our shared growth and understanding.

May this book reflect not just my dedication to changing narratives around Diet Culture, but also the profound gratitude and love I hold for you all, the unsung heroes of this journey.

With all my love and deepest appreciation.

PREFACE

Once upon a time, there was a young girl named Abigail. As a young child, she was a picky eater, and this upset her mom. Her mom made her feel guilty for leaving food uneaten, so Abigail always ate everything on her plate—no matter how hungry or full she was. Once she became a teenager, Abigail started to gain weight. The extra weight made her a target for other kids' comments and teasing at school. So, she went to her "skinny" friends for help. They were constantly talking about what foods they ate and avoided. It seemed to Abigail that dieting was the only way to be accepted by her peers and end the bullying. She decided to diet too. For a while, dieting worked. But at some point, it stopped working for her. For years, she tried every new diet that came out, hoping to find the one that would help her keep the weight off.

Even after she became an adult, she continued to feel the pressure to be thin. She felt that being overweight was causing her to lose opportunities for promotions at work and dating opportunities with men. The harder she tried to lose weight, the more disappointed she was by the results. No matter what she did, she could not seem to lose the weight she wanted or keep off what she lost. On top of that, she was exhausted, mentally and physically, by the endless cycle of strict dieting, hunger pangs, and bouts of low energy. She felt like she was fighting a losing battle. And she was.

Abigail began blaming herself, thinking if only she had more willpower, she could achieve her best weight. Her self-esteem plummeted. She struggled with terrible cravings that left her binging on sweets, cakes, and potato chips. Finally, dejected, she could take it no more.

Abigail reached out to me for help. There had to be a better way. And there was.

> There had to be a better way. And there was.

INTRODUCTION

We have learned more about the human body and its reaction to dieting in the last ten years than in the previous thousand, and we are learning more every day. What is now clear is that evolution has hardwired the human body to protect us from deprivation, which most popular diets include in some form or another. Scientific research has reliably shown that the body makes chemical and hormonal changes to counter the effects of deprivation, making weight loss by dieting extremely difficult to sustain.

My name is Dr. Supatra Tovar. I am one of the only clinical psychologists who is also a registered dietitian and fitness expert. I have spent years earning degrees in nutritional science and psychology to figure out how the mind and body are programmed to protect us and how they naturally work together against the main principles of most diets. But I did not learn these lessons easily.

Growing up, I was an active and athletic kid who never had to worry about weight or shape. I ate whatever I wanted, whenever I wanted, and never gained weight. I did not track calories or worry about the nutritional content of my food. Once I reached my late twenties, however, all of this changed. I started to gain weight, which was distressing to me. My carefree days of eating what I wanted when I wanted seemed to be over, and I was afraid of being ridiculed for being overweight. So I turned to the internet and to best-selling books and learned the "secrets" to losing weight. Most of the information out there stated that the only way to lose weight was to restrict my eating and to exercise excessively. So, I followed this advice. I became a Pilates instructor, massively upped my cardio, and restricted my eating. To my relief, it worked—for a while. Like most people, I eventually found myself back in the same place—feeling disappointed in myself for not staying disciplined enough. I realized I was trapped in a diet hamster wheel, and it was time for me to get off. I decided to learn more about nutrition and exercise, so I made some big life changes. I went to graduate school to study nutritional science and became a registered dietitian. After that, I earned my doctoral degree as a clinical psychologist. Having completed a thesis, much research, and a dissertation to boot, all I can say is that what I discovered was, at the very least, eye-opening.

Once I came to understand the reality of the body's negative reaction to dieting, I made it my goal to develop a better method for achieving and maintaining optimal health that did not go against the natural protective instincts of my body and my mind. I then devised a system based on the results of my research, my work on myself, and my extensive sessions with my clients. My system helps people who have grown weary of unsuccessful dieting create a long-term, sustainable way to achieve their healthiest self. My clients' successes inspired me to create my holistic health educational company ANEW, which stands for Advanced Nutrition and Emotional Wellness.

This book presents an overview of everything I have learned about psychology and the food we eat and how to work with, and not against, the body to naturally return to your healthiest weight. I know my approach truly works, and I want to share it with you.

This book will teach you the first few steps to follow to begin eliminating Diet Culture's horrible and negative influence while reshaping your relationship with yourself and your food. You will read stories of my clients (names and identifying details have been changed to protect confidentiality) and see how my system improved their circumstances for the better. This information will save you copious amounts of precious time and money by helping you understand the science of why diets are useless and tend to fail while providing you actionable, positive, and proactive steps to help you naturally achieve and maintain your optimal health. We will also return to Abigail's story at the end of the book so you can discover how Abigail deprogrammed herself from Diet Culture and learned how to trust *herself*. And by reading this book, so can you.

This book contains a little research-backed and validated science on psychology, a little science about your body, and a little science about nutrition—all of which I will translate and mix in with some good old common sense. Some of the terms may be new to you, so I have put many of them in bold and included a glossary in the back of the book for your reference. If you enjoy this book, I invite you to continue your journey toward your best self—healthy, self-confident, and at your natural weight—by taking my seven-module online course Deprogram Diet Culture. Taking the online course will help you go beyond this book and will solidify the information so you can live diet-free for life. It worked for me. It worked for my clients. And I am confident it will work for you.

Let us begin!

Chapter 1

STOP THE DIET HAMSTER WHEEL

Introduction

This chapter covers three fundamental topics:

- Why diets do not work, no matter how many times you get on the diet hamster wheel or how hard you try
- How to begin to deprogram yourself out of Diet Culture
- How to begin to reprogram yourself to focus on body positivity

By the end of this chapter, you will see how dieting sends most of us down a path toward failure, trapping us in an endless cycle of loss and regain. You will learn how getting off this hamster wheel puts you on a path toward loving and listening to your body so you can naturally achieve optimum physical and mental health.

Section 1: Why Diets Do Not Work

Samantha was unhappy with her weight. She had tried every diet under the sun, and yet she could not seem to lose the excess pounds that had been haunting her for years. She was determined to achieve the body she always wanted, so she kept pushing forward. She started out with the popular fad diets and even tried the ones that promised miraculous results in a short period of time.

No matter what she did, the weight kept coming back. She began to feel like she was fighting an uphill battle, and she was getting discouraged. She tried to stay motivated by thinking about how great it would feel to finally have the body of her dreams. She started to exercise more and make healthier food choices, but those efforts seemed to be in vain. She even struggled with periods of binging in between diets.

Every time she had some success, her weight loss would not last. She would always gain back the few pounds she had lost. She felt like she was stuck in an endless cycle of loss and regain, and she was frustrated. She had tried all the diets, from low carb to low fat, and nothing seemed to work. She was beginning to lose hope, and she was about to give up completely on dieting.

Finally, Samantha had enough. She came to me for help getting off the endless diet hamster wheel.

The Diet Hamster Wheel

If you ask any doctor, dietitian, fitness trainer, or person on the street how to lose weight, their most likely response will be, "Eat less, move more!" Then they will point you to the latest deprivation diet, one that requires you to cut out an entire food group as a way to reduce your calories significantly.

You have probably been told that consuming fewer calories and increasing your physical activity will lead to weight loss. Often, these diets initially work—after a period of suffering and deprivation, you lose some weight. But once you "cheat" or go off the diet, you end up regaining the weight you lost or gaining even more weight than before. Then you feel defeated, humiliated, and ashamed. Eventually, you find another deprivation diet to try, thinking, "I know this one is going to work!"

Then what happens?

The same situation as before—rinse and repeat.

This is what I call the diet hamster wheel. You are on a continuous cycle of diet and weight gain. You never achieve your goal, and often you gain more weight with each cycle. But before I explain how this happens, I'll discuss why it happens.

(Warning: we are going to explore some research-backed and validated science about nutrition and the body [citations included so you can check out the research]; but do not worry, I'll explain the science in an accessible and understandable way.)

Post-Starvation Fat Overshooting

When you repeatedly cycle through diets, many bodily processes ensure that the diet is unsuccessful. No matter your age, activity level, beginning BMI, or overall physical health, dieting to lose weight increases the chances of gaining weight and becoming more prone to obesity.[1] But why is that the case?

This is due to **post-starvation fat overshooting**, a phenomenon directed by the sympathetic nervous system that considers body weight, food intake, and body composition as determinants of what weight will be regained over the body's original weight set point after significant weight loss. You see, when you go on a diet, your body interprets the lack of food as starvation. In response, it attempts to convert fat and lean muscle tissue into the energy it needs. In doing so, your body relies on two independent control systems.

One system, the **body energy partitioning system,** considers the ratio of fat to lean muscle tissue the individual person has at the beginning of the diet. This system is controlled by our **sympathetic nervous system** (our survival fight-or-flight nervous system) and remembers the proportions of fat and lean muscle lost during the diet. The body is designed to survive by minimizing and resisting these losses, and this system works to replenish what was lost in the *same proportion* before the diet was followed.[2]

This is an important point. If you lose a combination of lean muscle and fat during your diet, your body's systems are designed *to regain both in the same ratio they were in before they were lost*. If you lose 5 pounds of lean muscle and 10 pounds of fat (for a 2:1 ratio), then when you regain 4 pounds of lean muscle, your body will maintain the same ratio and work to add 8 pounds of fat.

Your body cannot understand what your intentions are when you decide to go on a diet; it only knows that it is not receiving the same amounts or types of food it is used to. Your body goes into survival mode and pushes to regain what was lost as fast as it can.

The second system, **adaptive thermogenesis,** is controlled by the fat stores themselves. Thermogenesis means the *production of heat*; the heat is created when the body burns off fat stores. When you are dieting, you are providing your body with less food than it is used to. This triggers your body's survival mechanism, causing it to go into starvation mode as it perceives the lack of food as a pending danger. This kick-starts a second process called **suppressed thermogenesis** in which your body goes into a state of preservation, slows down metabolism, and inhibits fat loss.[3] You may believe that persistent dieting and exercising will continue to reduce your fat reserves, but in reality, your fat stores are becoming more resilient and working to resist your efforts. Moreover, after you stop dieting, your body is in recovery mode from what it perceived as a danger to its survival. To recover what was lost and return to a pre-threat state, the body will overcompensate and further decrease the rate of fat burning.

Why is that?

First, due to the protective systems mentioned above, the human body tends to interpret dieting as starvation and as a danger to our health. The body is designed to maintain a proportion of fat at the level it is accustomed to. As such, the body is programmed to resist sustained fat loss. In other words, the body is programmed to reject a new weight because that new weight has proportionally less fat than the body had before the diet started. When dieting is stopped, the body will attempt to return to its previous proportions. Unfortunately, the battle between the body and dieting efforts usually ultimately results in an overcorrection, *weight gain.*

How do our efforts to lose weight lead us to regain it? It is due to **compensatory hyperphagia.** Compensatory = to make up for what was lost before. Hyper = lots. Phagia = eat. To make up for what you lost when dieting, you may eat more, and sometimes even a significant amount more. In fact, the amount of fat and lean muscle you lose is inversely and independently correlated to the amount you might eat after dieting.

This is important because your body's instincts to protect you cause you to eat more than usual after a diet. Your body prioritizes restoring the fat you lost and adding back lean muscle while compensating for the energy deficit. Your body is constantly monitoring the amount of fat and lean muscle you lose, as well as the number of calories you omit due to your diet. All these variables factor in to how much you might overeat later.[4] Deprivation diets tend to be ineffective in the long run because the body, with its protective systems, and the mind, with its ambitions for weight loss, are not in sync. The lack of sustained results then creates a feeling of defeat and failure and a repeat of the cycle.

> Deprivation diets tend to be ineffective in the long run because the body, with its protective systems, and the mind, with its ambitions for weight loss, are not in sync.

This is why Samantha could not lose weight despite all her best efforts. She was fighting against her own body's survival mechanisms, which ensured that each diet would fail.

This is the diet hamster wheel. Exhausting, is it not? Why do we put ourselves on this endless, harmful hamster wheel? The answer lies in how we have become conditioned.

In the following section, we will investigate how societal standards regarding body image have shifted over time to what is now the ideal—with thinness and even emaciation as the goal. We will also examine the detrimental effects of today's social expectations and discuss ways to create a healthier and more sustainable outlook for yourself and your body.

Section 2: Deprogramming Diet Culture

After Samantha learned the science of why diets tend to fail, we began to explore all the influences that drew her to dieting in the first place.

Samantha examined the world around her. Everywhere she looked, she saw messages about beauty and the perfect body. From her parents' comments about how she should eat less and exercise more, to the seemingly endless photos of perfect bodies on her social media feeds, to all her friends who were skinny no matter what they ate, Samantha was constantly reminded she was not thin.

No matter how hard she tried to resist, the pressure to be skinny was overwhelming. She felt like she was constantly judged and never good enough. She was so uncomfortable with her body that she avoided activities, events, and seeing friends in person. She spent more and more time online. She believed that being skinny was the only way to fit in and be accepted in real life.

Why Do We Diet?

We have grown up in an environment that encourages us to diet to look like the idealized images of male and female supermodels. The basis for these images and the impacts they have on us are based on our biases.

LOOKISM

Lookism is a bias that causes us to focus solely upon physical appearance. First, we make judgments about a person based on their physical looks and form our opinion of them without any other information. These judgments then influence the way we interact with them, and we often favor people who are deemed more attractive over those who are seen as not attractive.[5]

WEIGHTISM

Weightism is an even more insidious form of prejudice hidden beneath the surface of Lookism. Weightism is bias and discrimination against those who are considered overweight or obese. Weightism is considered to be as prominent as racism or sexism but is more widely accepted than both.[6] Weightism is perpetuated by the constant reinforcement of negative stereotypes that portray people of larger body sizes as being lazy, unintelligent, incompetent, and disorganized.[7]

A closer inspection of history reveals that the connection between Weightism and its prejudices have changed over time. Before the 1900s, plumpness was seen as an indication of wealth and health in both Europe and America. Poor people were usually very thin due to the physical demands of labor and the lack of affordable food. On the other side of the social spectrum, wealthy people enjoyed higher-calorie meals and more sedentary lifestyles. And although those meals usually had higher levels of fat, they were overall more nutritious than the foods available to the poorer members of society. This led to the belief that being overweight resulted in greater immunity against the diseases that ravaged society at the time. In hindsight, the stark discrepancy in the life expectancies of the wealthy and poor had as much to do with access to health care as it had to do with nutritious foods. Nevertheless, these social disparities led to the predominant belief of the time that it was more preferable to be plump than not.

At the beginning of the 1900s, people's outlooks shifted dramatically. A variety of foods once only accessible to the wealthy became widely available to the public. The Industrial Revolution led to less physically demanding labor. And as people became less gaunt, the affluent ones in society no longer considered it desirable to be overweight. The wealthy began to adopt a new dietary regimen to create a distinct body type, thereby distinguishing themselves from the rest of society.[8] From that point on, plumpness was viewed as a manifestation of an individual's lack of will to succeed or as an indication of their moral and personal deficiencies. For women, the hourglass figure became the new ideal to strive for. This was the dawn of **Diet Culture**.

Today, it has been found through research that Weightism, or fat shaming, is frequently experienced in many contexts, such as workplaces, health-care centers, educational institutions, and other areas of society.[9] The media, along with our family, friends, peers, and society, have made it common for us to feel pressure to conform to certain body standards.[10] Our prejudices contribute to the promotion of Diet Culture, which is the drive to achieve the ideal physical form.

If you use social media, watch TV, read magazines, or overhear conversations at work or school, you will likely observe both Lookism and Weightism. This can be seen in the clothes people purchase, the plastic surgery and skin treatments they get, the weight-loss medication they vie to purchase, and especially in the food they choose to eat. Advertisements are crafted to make you believe that you are inadequate and must do something to achieve the "perfect" standard.

> By accepting Diet Culture, you are likely to waste money on superfluous items, undergo invasive surgeries, take weight-loss medication, and live permanently in a state of dissatisfaction.

What is the cost of this pursuit? Starvation or elimination dieting is not beneficial for your mental, physical, emotional, or financial health. By accepting Diet Culture, you are likely to waste money on superfluous items, undergo invasive surgeries, take weight-loss medication, and live permanently in a state of dissatisfaction. Furthermore, as mentioned in the prior section, engaging in starvation or extreme dieting will likely cause you to gain back any weight you have lost and become stuck in a perpetual cycle of dieting.

Have you had enough? I know I have, and I know Samantha has! But we can change this situation.

How to Deprogram Yourself from Diet Culture

Deprogramming yourself involves three steps:

1. Clean your social media feed.
2. Limit advertising consumption.
3. Reduce contact with toxic people.

CLEAN YOUR SOCIAL MEDIA FEED

Start your social media cleanup by examining your current Instagram, Facebook, TikTok, and YouTube feeds. Scrutinize the accounts you follow and ask yourself what you see and how you feel when you look at social media. If your response is negative, such as "terrible," "I hate myself," or "I am too fat," it is time to clean up your feed. I did this with Samantha, and she was shocked to see that most of her feed was straight out of Diet Culture. Do we need to see it? NO! We are much happier when we do not! Samantha learned this quickly.

To create a positive, uplifting environment, we should hide, block, or unfollow anyone or anything that causes us to feel any negative emotions. This way, we can promote a more supportive atmosphere and remove any influences that may be holding us back.

LIMIT ADVERTISEMENT CONSUMPTION

The next step is to stop subscribing to all fashion or entertainment magazines and stop watching advertisements on TV. Streaming services give us more control over what we see than ever before. Have you ever felt like you were not good enough after seeing an advertisement? Many ads are designed to make us feel inferior or inadequate, leading us to think that we need to buy something to fill a void. But if you take a step back and notice what is really going on, you will see that these ads are simply trying to get you to buy something by making you feel worse about yourself.

Advertising is designed to manipulate you and make you feel like you need something that you do not. It is meant to pressure you into spending your hard-earned money on something you do not really need. Avoiding these sources of negativity is the simplest and quickest way to remove their damaging effects from your life. Samantha began evaluating the ads that filled her feed and realized how much they were influencing her mental health. Hiding these ads and limiting social media time helped her regain her self-esteem.

This is not about completely cutting yourself off from the world. This is about finding the most straightforward way to achieve success by surrounding yourself with inspirational people and media and breaking away from any negative beliefs you may have. This is about surrounding yourself with positivity and deprogramming your mind!

REDUCE CONTACT WITH TOXIC PEOPLE

This step is much more difficult. Examine the people in your life, including friends and colleagues. Do you have unhealthy relationships with some of them? Do you feel worse about yourself after spending time with certain people? Are you being pressured to diet or exercise by someone? It is especially crucial that you set limits for yourself when you are engaging in self-improvement to restore your physical and mental well-being. The physical symptoms you experience when around these toxic relationships can be telling; you may get a headache, feel tension in your neck and shoulders, or get a bad feeling in the pit of your stomach. Overall, you likely feel worse about yourself after spending time with them.

If you find yourself in the presence of someone toxic, consider creating boundaries to limit your exposure to them.

Instead, focus on spending time with people who make you feel good, promote healthy habits, and accept you unconditionally. Samantha realized that some people in her life were negative influences, and she limited the time she spent with them while she increased the time she spent with the fun and positive people in her life. This made a huge difference in how she felt.

You can usually tell when you meet positive, good people. They tend to have an air of lightness about them and often wear a smile and say kind words. When you are with them, you may feel uplifted, and you may leave their company feeling better about yourself. I hope you surround yourself with people who support you as you break free from Diet Culture and begin to reprogram your mind for health, joy, and freedom from cycling through diets.

Section 3: Reprogramming a Path to a Healthier You

Throughout the course of our work together, Samantha began to understand that beauty comes in all shapes and sizes and in many different forms. She was encouraged to look past other people's ideas of beauty and to embrace her own uniqueness. Samantha's perspective shifted over time. She realized how misguided the pursuit to be skinny was and that she could be accepted just the way she was. She began to embrace her body and the things that made her unique, and she worked to stop comparing herself to others. She started to take better care of herself and to focus on the things that made her happy. Paradoxically, once she focused on listening to and honoring herself, she naturally lost weight without dieting, simply by finding movement that brought her joy and by listening to her body's cues to eat and stop eating. Samantha was finally able to appreciate her own beauty and accept herself for who she was. With newfound confidence, she was able to be her authentic self, and she felt more connected to her friends and the world around her. She realized that beauty is not defined by a number on the scale—it is about feeling confident and loving yourself.

> Beauty comes in all shapes and sizes and in many different forms.

This section will explain how to replace the negative influences in your life and reprogram your mind to have a more positive outlook, leading you toward a healthier lifestyle. It is normal to feel overwhelmed by the process of reprogramming your mind and entering unfamiliar territory. We'll take it step by step.

Repopulate Your Social Media Feed

To begin the process of reprogramming your mind, start by refilling your social media feed with positive and uplifting content. Find websites or social media profiles that make you feel happy and inspired. Next, review your subscription lists and favorites. Prioritize the ones that make you feel good or happy. Surrounding yourself with positive content is so much better than subjecting yourself to weight stigmatization. Weight stigmatization can cause a series of problems such as the ones in this list developed by Natasha A. Schvey and colleagues:[11]

- Increased depression
- Damaged self-esteem
- **Negative perfectionism** (or the unhappy pursuit of the thin ideal)
- **Body dysmorphia** (or the perception that certain parts of your body are larger than they are)
- Poor body image
- Higher risk of suicidality
- Increase in eating disorders

- Unhealthy eating behaviors, increased loss of control while eating, binge eating, eating in secret, and avoidance of exercise

> To begin the process of reprogramming your mind, start by refilling your social media feed with positive and uplifting content.

Once you take this step, almost all social media sites will recommend other sites based on your choices. Rather than seeing an endless feed of Diet Culture, you could be seeing an endless feed of content that makes you happy.

Body Positivity

Rooted in positive psychology, the concept of **body positivity** focuses on promoting psychological resilience, health, self-compassion, and empathy while also embracing a more inclusive and positive view of body image.[12] Researchers commonly define body positivity as an overarching love and respect for the body. Body positivity typically includes the following:

- Appreciate, admire, and accept the unique beauty of the body and the functions that it performs, even if those aspects are inconsistent with idealized images.
- Feel comfortable and happy with your body, which is often reflected as confidence and an outer radiance, or a "glow."

- Interpret incoming information in a body-protective manner whereby most positive information is internalized and most negative information is rejected or reframed.[13]

The body positivity movement includes a concept of beauty that minimizes the importance of perceived imperfections and rejects negative media.[14] Having an appreciation for your body and seeing the beauty within yourself leads to improved body image. This is not only the foundation for behaviors that boost your joy, such as more self-compassion and empathy, but it can also help you defend against feelings of depression and anxiety. Samantha learned how to do this. And so can you.

> Having an appreciation for your body and seeing the beauty within yourself leads to improved body image.

So far in this chapter, we have learned a lot. A short review is in order because these concepts serve as the basis for the rest of our work:

- The collective belief is that to lose weight, you need to eat less and exercise more.
- Weight loss through deprivation dieting seems simple but is never easy to sustain.
- The goal is to have your body work with your ambitions, not against you.

- The media pushes a certain body type as the ideal, bombards you with images to reinforce that idea, and tries to sell you various diets that change every two to three years, trapping you in an endless cycle of deprivation.

Over time, exercise has become a larger component of Diet Culture's formula for weight loss. Social media and advertising are laced with images of fit bodies sweating profusely, overtly linking a dedication to exercise as a measure of an individual's determination and sacrifice to achieve the ideal weight. What we have not yet discussed is how exercise can worsen the detrimental effects of Diet Culture.

Exercise Should Not Be Punishment

The promotion of punishing exercise regimens as the way to obtain the ideal figure has become increasingly relentless and difficult to avoid. Movie promotions use extremely fit movie stars headlining superhero and action movies to highlight the exercises, the eating routines, the sacrifice, and the dedication leading up to each debut. The ambition to look and feel like the heroes of the big screen can push anyone toward compulsive behaviors and the urge to take unnecessary risks with their health. I met many of my Pilates clients when they were fed up with exercise that did not bring them joy or make them feel good. They complained of exercises that left them in pain and discomfort for days. These clients were seeking an alternative to punishing workouts. This is the same sentiment that Samantha relayed to me. To lose weight, Samantha tried

CrossFit and reported to me that this punishing form of exercise always left her feeling exhausted and depleted.

After taking a closer look at what goes on behind the scenes of celebrities' exercise regimens, a less-than-ideal picture emerges. To achieve the physiques seen on the screen, many celebrities undertake a strenuous six- to eight-hour training schedule every day. These workouts may be combined with performance-enhancing drugs or weight-loss medications that alter the body's chemistry.

For most people, including celebrities, maintaining this type of exercise regimen for more than a few weeks or months is not realistic and can be detrimental in the long run. In fact, the toll of this type of training can be physical as well as psychological. Many who attempt to sustain this level of exercise end up with physical injuries, nutritional deficiencies, and other serious consequences. On the mental health side, research has demonstrated that engaging in too much punishing physical activity can result in **appearance anxiety** (being excessively concerned about one's physical appearance), body dysmorphia (feeling that certain parts of the body are bigger than they actually are), the development of eating disorders, and low self-esteem.[15] Other studies show that engaging in too much exercise can also result in **negative affect** and perfectionism, compulsive tendencies, negative emotions, and a tendency to socially isolate.[16] When Samantha was doing CrossFit, she complained of many of these same ill effects.

Many of these training regimens are often paired with drugs like Ozempic or Wegovy for that extra edge in the fight for weight loss. It is important to know that these drugs are tweaking the body's natural systems by slowing digestion and suppressing appetite. These weight-loss medications can have unpleasant and dangerous side effects as well, such as nausea, gastrointestinal distress, or even gastrointestinal paralysis, headaches, and dizziness. In addition, these drugs can result in malnourishment if proper nutrition is not maintained. Using these drugs can lead to physical and mental health difficulties and, at the very least, make it hard to concentrate and perform daily functions. Moreover, the results of these drugs are usually only sustainable while using them; when celebrities and the public stop taking them, the weight they lost often comes back. This cause-and-effect can create a mental and physical reliance on the drugs to suppress the body's natural systems and lead individuals to take them indefinitely to maintain the weight loss.

Some people are willing to go to extreme lengths to maintain their physical appearance. But you may be looking for a way to sustain your body without the use of costly drugs and surgery. On this path, you will avoid the pitfalls often experienced by people who feel compelled to exercise excessively, undergo surgery, or take weight-loss medications to shed pounds. This is what Samantha started to learn.

As a psychologist dedicated to maximizing mental health, I strongly suggest to my clients that they take pleasure in their exercise routine. You do not need to push yourself to the point where you are too tired or are in pain the rest of the day; exercise should not be a punishment.

Exercising in a healthy way is not just good for your physical body—it can leave you with an emotional boost, too! Endorphins are the feel-good chemicals that are released when you exercise, resulting in a happy and satisfied feeling. If you are feeling a strong sense of accomplishment and satisfaction after a workout, then you know you are doing it right! Healthy exercise can help boost resilience to depression and anxiety while also providing you with a sense of joy and delight from your physical activity.

> Healthy exercise can help boost resilience to depression and anxiety while also providing you with a sense of joy and delight from your physical activity.

Generally, exercise forms such as yoga and Pilates are excellent for reducing stress. These types of restorative exercises rely on mindful breathing, where each exercise or pose is accompanied by conscious inhalation and exhalation. By engaging in restorative exercise, which combines breathing techniques with muscle strengthening and stretching, you can experience a plethora of beneficial stress-reduction results such as decreased depression and anxiety, reduced inflammation and cortisol production, and increased mental health and self-worth. This is the type of practice that Samantha adopted, and she reported an increase in energy, mental clarity, and an improvement in mood by starting her Pilates practice.

Discovering the ideal form of exercise for you is a personal process. It should be based on how you feel after doing it. You'll know you are headed in the right direction if you can say, "Wow, I feel great!" or "That made me so happy!" Please note, it is always important to consult a medical professional to get the recommendations that are right for you. Exercise does not have to be a punishment for last night's meal. It can be a sustainable, healthy way to increase energy, longevity, and stamina. If Samantha could find her way past punishing forms of exercise, then so can you!

Chapter 2

REDEFINING YOUR IDEAL FOOD RELATIONSHIP

Introduction

In this chapter, we will delve into the way you relate to food and how you can achieve the relationship with food you always wanted. We focus on three fundamental topics:

- Analyzing your childhood relationship with food
- Examining your present relationship with food
- Learning how to stop vilifying your food

We will talk about the marketing tactics food companies use to convince you to buy their products. We will also discuss your past experiences to gain awareness about your present relationship with food.

By the end of this chapter, you will see how your earliest associations with food paved the way for an unhealthy present relationship with food. Once you become aware of these influences, you can shape the relationship into the one you want to have.

Section 1: Examine Your Childhood Relationship with Food

Esperanza is a young woman who sought help with binge eating. Growing up poor, Esperanza was told by her parents that she could never be sure when or where her next meal would be. She would often eat whatever she could whenever she could, and sometimes she would eat large quantities to delay the next hunger cycle as much as possible. She carried these habits into adulthood, even when she no longer lived in poverty. Esperanza tried to control her binge eating with various diets and exercise regimens, but nothing seemed to work. She felt embarrassed and ashamed of this, and she was reluctant to seek professional help. When she finally decided to call me, she was surprised to find out how common her symptoms were. I guided her through one of her first tasks, which was to gain insight into her past eating behaviors so she could reshape her current behaviors.

When I start working with clients to help them break away from Diet Culture, I thoroughly examine the eating habits they formed when they were growing up. I cannot overemphasize how crucial it is to understand your past and your connection to food. Most of my clients have never reflected on their childhoods or recalled the events that influenced their dietary behaviors. Conscious awareness of those experiences or not, those events and memories are often at the root of our issues with eating.

Most of my clients recall having an intuitive approach to eating when they were younger; they would eat when they were hungry and stop when they were full. This is a natural and organic way of eating. Most young children tune in to their body's signals to decide when and how much to eat. As we grow up, these instincts are muted as we are exposed to influences inside and outside our homes.

External Influences

Commercials have an immense impact on people, particularly when it comes to food. Children are especially susceptible to such influences, and these formative experiences remain with us well into adulthood.

With the consumer food market worth around $8 trillion, it is not surprising to discover that companies spend a lot of money to make money. The food industry hires scientists to identify the ingredients that make food products more appealing to customers. Knowing which ingredients can lead to greater sales is a key part of these food companies' strategies to capture as much of the market as possible. In addition, the food industry pays advertising agencies large sums of money to influence consumers' buying habits. Nevertheless, even though advertising and commercials are enormously influential, the most important influence comes from the home.

Internal Influences

What do you remember about your family meals? What was your childhood eating style?

- Did you all sit at the table together?
- Did you all eat on TV trays in front of the TV?
- Did you eat any meals together?
- Did you routinely eat at a certain time every day whether you were hungry or not?
- If you did eat a family meal at the dinner table, did your family encourage you to eat until you were way past satisfied and overfull?
- Did your parents tell you or force you to eat everything on your plate?
- Did they use guilt to force you to clean your plate by telling you about starving children across the world?
- Were you already full and just got fuller and more uncomfortable so you could "earn" dessert?

How you grew up shaped and formed your present coping mechanisms and eating styles. As a child, you absorbed the patterns of your family unit. Today, you model in your adult life what you observed in your home growing up. One of the strongest influences on your life is the relationship bond with your primary caregivers, which is referred to as the type of attachment that the individual develops. The term *attachment* is derived from **attachment theory**, developed by psychologist John Bowlby, which explains how the very first relationships you form with your primary caregivers influence the methods we adopt for coping and the possible development of eating problems.

> How you grew up shaped and formed your present coping mechanisms and eating styles.

Think about the impact of the messages you received as a child. As an adult, you may not realize how those nicknames or comments from family and friends—often said in jest or with the best of intentions—greatly shaped the way you think about yourself and your food. You don't think about how your parents were teaching you to diet as you watched them diet. You also don't realize how the food environment in which you grew up shaped the way you eat as an adult. As you can see with Esperanza, she was told that food was scarce, so she learned to eat whatever she could, whenever she could, in case there would not be another meal for a very long time. Gaining insight into these powerful childhood messages helped her develop self-awareness.

When you were young, you naturally had a mindful style of eating. You ate when you were hungry, you stopped when you had eaten enough, you did not eat things you did not like, and happily ate things you did like. Then the collective impact of all the influences I have mentioned overwhelmed you, muffled your instincts, and reshaped your relationship with food.

In the next section, we will examine how our relationship to food evolved into what it is today. When we gain awareness of our choices and motivations to eat and learn how to distinguish the physical and emotional cues to eat, we can begin to rebuild this relationship into something healthier and ultimately more satisfying.

Section 2: Examine Your Present Relationship with Food

Let us see how Esperanza's childhood eating affected her adult life. As you recall, Esperanza grew up in poverty and always felt as if she was on the edge of starvation. As she grew older, this relationship with food morphed into a self-soothing mechanism—a comfort cloak she would wrap around herself in the face of emotional pain and stress. Every stressful encounter, life difficulty, or relationship problem sent her spiraling into the comforting arms of food. This coping mechanism eventually evolved into mindless binge eating whenever she felt upset.

Eating helped to numb the pain temporarily, but it never truly healed her wounds. She consumed vast amounts of food without realizing it, almost as if on autopilot, with her mind often elsewhere, fixated on the emotional turmoil she was experiencing. This mindless binge eating, however, was more than a cry for help; it was Esperanza's silent rebellion against her stressful past, an attempt to reclaim control and find a sense of inner peace that was otherwise denied to her.

Esperanza's story may be a personal journey, but it is a tale that resonates with many who have sought refuge in food to cope with emotional pain. It is a crucial reminder of how issues from childhood can significantly impact your relationship with food and shape your behavioral patterns later in life. Esperanza courageously navigated her path toward healing by understanding how her past dictated her current relationship with food. And so can you.

In this section, you will focus on your current relationship with food. This requires cultivating an awareness of your eating habits, and this awareness may initially feel unfamiliar. Over the course of time, this awareness may have been eclipsed by unhealthy eating behaviors that cause you to eat mechanically or mindlessly. Alternatively, your awareness may have been obscured by emotional eating. Or a combination of both factors may be at play. We'll examine these two eating styles below.

Mindless Eating

As the phrase implies, **mindless eating** is when we eat in a distracted environment without conscious awareness of or attention to our food. Later in this book we are going to learn its opposite, mindful eating. But before we do, we need to examine why mindless eating is harming your health, causing you to overeat, and disconnecting you from your emotions.

Fundamentally, mindless eating entails a disregard for the body's inherent hunger and satiety signals because our attention is elsewhere. The common consequence of mindless eating is that we end up eating when not genuinely hungry, or we ignore the body's signals of being full, continuing to eat beyond our needs. Such behaviors not only increase the risk of weight gain and related health complications, but may also pave the way for suppressed emotions and potential mental health disorders.

> The more distracted we are, the more likely we are to eat well beyond our needs.

A 2013 study by researchers Jane Ogden and others[1] delved into the effects of various distractions on eating habits. Participants were randomly assigned to one of four conditions of distracted eating: while driving, during social interaction, when alone, or while watching television. The findings revealed that the food intake of all participants was not in sync with their actual hunger levels, indicating a pattern of eating even when not hungry. Furthermore, the study revealed that eating while driving and during social interactions heightened the likelihood of eating past the point of satiety more significantly than while watching television or eating alone.[2] In short, this study implies that the more distracted we are, the more likely we are to eat well beyond our needs.

Emotional Eating

Emotional eating, as you might gather from the term itself, refers to situations when our emotions significantly influence our eating habits. One form of this, as Esperanza experienced, is comfort eating. This happens when we are dealing with feelings of anxiety, stress, or sadness, which can make us gravitate toward foods usually high in fat and carbohydrates—the kind that can bring us a sense of warmth and solace. Another example of emotional eating from Esperanza's experience is binge eating, where she consumed considerably more food than usual in one sitting. This behavior is typically associated with negative emotions like anger, stress, sadness, shame, guilt, jealousy, hopelessness, or frustration.

A different study, by Allan Geliebter and Angela Aversa in 2003,[3] explored how the eating styles of those considered underweight and overweight were affected when confronted with negative emotions. Their findings indicated that those considered underweight usually ate less when grappling with negative emotional states, while those considered overweight tended to eat more.[4] Additionally, in a result that surprised no one who has eaten too much during a holiday dinner, both groups in that study reported eating more when experiencing positive emotional states. Remember picking your elastic-waisted outfit based on your eventual post-Thanksgiving food coma?

From a young age, we develop coping mechanisms, such as our eating styles, to help us through emotional or stressful times. Feeling stressed, sad, or anxious can cause either an increase or decrease in food intake. Some may cope with depression or anxiety by shutting down and not eating, while others may cope by reaching for the nearest quart of ice cream. And we also learn how to eat by modeling the behaviors of those around us.

> Some may cope with depression or anxiety by shutting down and not eating, while others may cope by reaching for the nearest quart of ice cream.

> ### Mindless and Emotional Eating Exercise
>
> To help determine whether you eat mindlessly or emotionally, because of being distracted, because of routine, because of emotion, or because you are hungry, start by remembering yesterday's dinner. Think about the time and setting in which you ate.
>
> - What time was it?
> - Why did you eat at that time?
> - Were you hungry?
> - What were you feeling before you ate?
> - What did you eat?
> - How much did you eat?
> - How did you feel when you were eating?
> - What was the setting in which you ate?
> - Was your attention distracted in any way?
> - How did you feel afterward?
> - Did you feel hungry, full, or overfull after?
>
> Asking yourself these simple questions is a way to start developing self-awareness, which is invaluable in gaining insight into why you might eat when you are not physiologically hungry.

I hope you are finding more awareness about any unhelpful coping mechanisms you might have formed, such as mindless and emotional eating. By cultivating awareness about your current relationship to food, you can begin to change this relationship to a healthier one. But before we embark on that, it is important to examine our tendency to vilify our foods. That is what we will explore in the next section.

Section 3: Learn to Stop Vilifying Your Food

Before coming to see me, Esperanza's life cycled between dieting and binging that left her weighing more and feeling worse. After one particularly distressing and physically taxing binge, Esperanza took to the internet for help. She learned about "eating clean" and decided to try it.

She started by cutting out all processed foods, focusing more on fresh fruits and vegetables, whole grains, and lean proteins. At first, it seemed like a great idea, but soon Esperanza found herself becoming increasingly obsessed with what she was eating. She was counting calories, avoiding certain foods and ingredients, and obsessing over food labels to make sure she was eating the "right" things.

This food obsession and subsequent restriction worked for a while, until Esperanza could no longer take the restriction and went back to binging. This cycle of binging and restricting eventually led her to see me.

Esperanza was able to learn strategies—which we'll cover later in this book—to work through her stressful childhood binge-eating patterns. In time, Esperanza was able to regain control of her relationship with food. She was able to enjoy her meals again, without the guilt and overthinking that led to eventual binging. She was finally able to heal her relationship with food.

"Good" Food, "Bad" Food

You probably grew up learning the concepts of "good" and "bad" food long ago, perhaps even before you learned the concept of dieting. When you think of "good" food, what images come to mind? Now, when you think of "bad" food, what images come to mind?

What if I tell you that to kick Diet Culture to the curb, you need to drop these labels and adopt a neutral mindset—to think of food as just "food," neither good nor bad?

"But wait!" you cry. "You are a dietitian! Are you not always yelling at us about eating good food and avoiding bad foods?"

This is true. I will not deny it. Dietitians have the word "diet" in their name for a reason. But the reason I am not a fan of labeling food as good or bad is because my experiences have shown me that to successfully reach our goals, we have to find the solutions that are the best for our bodies and our mental health. As we uncovered in the initial chapter, dieting can often be a path that leads to unhealthy and unproductive outcomes. Hence, for me, labeling food as good or bad would likely follow the same counterproductive lines. When we box food into such categories, it inadvertently leads to the demonization of certain types of food and makes the so-called "bad food" a forbidden food.

> What if I tell you that to kick Diet Culture to the curb, you need to drop these labels and adopt a neutral mindset—to think of food as just "food," neither good nor bad?

Let us take a quick stroll down memory lane and revisit the diet trends of the past; we will also examine those of the present. You will notice a recurring theme—most of the diets place certain ingredients or food groups in the bad or off-limits category. They tell us to eliminate those foods altogether or, at the very least, drastically reduce our consumption of those foods. In short, categorizing food rigidly can lead us down a slippery slope. Let us name a few of these diets:

- Carb-restriction or carb-elimination diets such as Atkins, keto, paleo, and South Beach
- Super low-calorie diets such as intermittent fasting, Body for Life, Cookie Diet, Nutrisystem, Weight Watchers, and Jenny Craig
- Crash diets like cabbage soup, Beverly Hills, and Subway diet
- Animal protein reduction or elimination via vegetarianism or veganism
- Detox and food-specific diets such as juice cleanse, Master Cleanse, Whole30, clean eating, and macrobiotics

The promotion of these diet plans tends to tap into our longing for quick fixes. They often label certain foods as fundamentally harmful and tell you that you need to deprive yourself of them. Think of these diets like buildings with unstable foundations. If you aspire to having physical and mental well-being, it is imperative that you focus on fortifying the foundation first. Adopting these diets could not only derail you from reaching your weight-loss objectives but could potentially invite more detrimental consequences.

It is crucial to remember that balance and mindfulness are the keys to a healthy relationship with food, not deprivation and extremism. If you choose to follow some of the extreme diets I have mentioned, you might find yourself spiraling down a path that encourages unhealthy behaviors and may even lead to the development of an eating disorder, some of which are listed below:

- **Anorexia nervosa** is characterized by extreme self-starvation, fear of gaining weight, extremely low body weight, and body dysmorphia (thinking of certain body parts as larger than they actually are).
- **Bulimia nervosa** is characterized by negative self-evaluation, binge eating larger than normal amounts of food in a discrete (two-hour) time period, lack of control over one's eating, and inappropriate and distressing methods to counteract the binge—like vomiting or over-exercising—at least one day per week for three months.
- **Binge eating disorder** is characterized by negative self-evaluation, binge eating larger than normal amounts of food in a discrete (two-hour) time period, lack of control over one's eating, and extreme distress over the binges at least one day per week for three months.[5]

Clean Eating

What exactly is **clean eating**? The generally accepted definition is eating food free from pesticides, additives, preservatives, and impurities. The foods are eaten in a way that promotes cleansing and purifying the body.[6] But even clean eating can be taken to an extreme.

You might ask why eating clean foods is a problem. Anything taken to an extreme is risky for you, and the clean eating approach is near the top of that slippery slope. The danger surrounding this diet is the aggressive hyperconsciousness that usually accompanies an obsession with eating only "pure" foods. As a result of this hyperconsciousness and the distress it eventually causes, we are now seeing a type of eating disorder called orthorexia nervosa.

Orthorexia Nervosa

According to a group of researchers led by Dr. Hellas Cena, an academic researcher from the University of Pavia in Italy, people suffering from **orthorexia nervosa** are obsessively preoccupied with healthy nutrition or reaching a certain body ideal to the point where it impairs their ability to have a positive social life, or it impacts their health and nutrition. They tend to take irrational actions to avoid "unhealthy" foods and seek organic, "pure," or "safe" foods. People suffering from orthorexia nervosa typically create a set of self-imposed nutritional rules or engage in highly ritualized, restrictive, and selective eating styles that lead them to experience emotional consequences—such as high levels of distress or anxiety.[7] It is important to note that orthorexia nervosa is not yet listed as an official eating disorder in the *Diagnostic and Statistical Manual of Mental Disorders*, though many researchers and clinicians agree it should be.

When the pursuit of eating healthy turns into an obsession, or when it leads to the complete elimination of foods like grains and starchy carbohydrates, things start to get dicey. If you choose to follow some of the extreme diets I have mentioned, you might find yourself spiraling down a path that encourages unhealthy behaviors and potentially even leads to the development of an eating disorder. Having spent numerous years studying and treating these disorders, I can vouch for the fact that they can significantly impact mental well-being. While eating disorders can be challenging to treat, it is important to remember that healing is always possible.

If you suspect that you may be dealing with one of these disorders, I strongly encourage you to seek out a highly trained and experienced therapist. They can provide invaluable guidance and support as you journey through the recovery process. You are not alone in this, and professional help can make a world of difference. I have seen how often Diet Culture's mindset and the demonization of certain foods lead to eating disorders. This inspired me to make it my mission to help my clients nip such harmful thought patterns in the bud, preventing the emergence of an eating disorder before it gets a chance to take root.

> I am a big advocate of the belief that NO FOOD should be strictly off limits.

When you free yourself from the shackles of Diet Culture, you start to see food for what it truly is—just food, free from any categorical labels. I am a big advocate of the belief that NO FOOD should be strictly off limits. This is because the moment you perceive something as being scarce or designate certain foods as forbidden or off limits, you start to view them as tantalizing temptations, something taboo or restricted. This mindset can make you crave those foods even more, leading you toward overindulgence or binge eating. You are tricked into thinking you can never eat those foods again, so you might as well consume as much as you can in one sitting. This way of thinking does not usually end well for most of us. It often leads to binging, feelings of guilt, shame, and self-reproach. This is not how you should be living—where is the joy in it? Trust me when I say it does not have to be like this.

How do you come to terms with the idea that there is no such thing as bad food and that nothing should be strictly off limits? The key lies in learning to listen—truly listen—to your body, to recognize and fulfill its natural needs. By tuning in, rather than checking out, your body can guide you, letting you know what it needs, when you are hungry, and when you have had enough. It is a return to your roots, a rekindling of the mindful eating habits you once had. You are going to relearn the art of listening to your body and start tuning out all the other distracting voices that cloud your mind. Life is too short not to enjoy food. Let us embark on this journey toward mindful eating together. This is what we will learn in the next chapter. This is what Esperanza learned.

Chapter 3

HUNGER AND FULLNESS VERSUS EMOTIONAL OR MINDLESS EATING

Introduction

This chapter will examine the steps you can take to remember how to listen to your body's hunger and fullness cues and distinguish them from emotional and mindless eating. We will focus on three fundamental objectives:

- Rediscovering hunger and fullness cues
- Learning to distinguish hunger and fullness from emotional and mindless eating
- Discussing unhealthy cravings and how they are tied to Diet Culture

At the end of this chapter, you will have a better understanding of your body's signals and how to resist succumbing to unhealthy cravings.

Section 1: Relearning about Hunger and Fullness

Ava was a young girl when her parents divorced. The shock of the split left her feeling an emptiness that she could not quite explain. It was like a part of her had been lost, and she did not know how to get it back. She felt alone and confused, and so she turned to food for comfort. At first, it was small treats—a piece of cake here, a cookie there. But soon she found herself searching more frequently for comfort in food. She would eat until she felt full, and then she would eat some more. Her overeating became a pattern—one that she was unable to break and that persisted into adolescence and adulthood. Ava had forgotten what true hunger and fullness felt like, and this affected her weight and her self-esteem. After her weight had reached a point where she felt no one would love her, she sought my help. We examined her childhood relationship with food to make the connections with her emotions and then began examining what true physiological hunger and fullness feels like.

In chapter 2, we learned how our past relationships, modeled behavior, and external influences shape our eating behaviors. We learned what emotional eating and mindless eating are, and we explored how the vilification of food can lead us to unhealthy thinking and to a subsequent lack of control that comes from creating taboo or off-limits foods. In this section, we are going to reconnect to our natural hunger and fullness cues and reprogram our thoughts to help us listen to those cues. We are going to rediscover what you already knew when you were six years old but may have forgotten.

As a child, you naturally possessed a keen instinct to listen to your body. At a tender age, most of us had yet to face the full brunt of societal, familial, and media influences that can push us away from our innate eating patterns.

Like Ava, these social and cultural influences gradually began to shape your behaviors, and you started to lose touch with the natural cues of your body. When your internal signals become drowned out and no longer guide your eating, you can find yourself searching for guidance from external sources. Diets become appealing, as they offer a straightforward framework: shun the bad food, embrace the good food, and witness the transformation. But as you immerse yourself in this structure, you slowly lose touch with the body's sensations of hunger and satiety.

How do you rediscover what you have left behind? The first step is to foster a degree of self-awareness. You can achieve this by mastering the art of self-regulation.

Self-Regulation

What is self-regulation?

Self-regulation is simply paying attention to yourself. Two researchers, Shauna Shapiro and Gary Schwartz, introduced the term when they discovered that receiving conscious feedback about your body increases your awareness and naturally regulates your system.[1] This applies to hunger and fullness because when you consciously tune in to your body, you find that your body provides you with natural physical cues to indicate whether you are hungry, satisfied, or full.

To be able to self-regulate, you first need to reacquaint yourself with the actual sensation of physical hunger. To achieve this, it is important to fully comprehend what hunger truly means.

Hunger

Hunger can be defined as a metabolic state that arises due to a deficiency of nutrients or energy. It is typically marked by a driving motivation or an expressed need to consume food. This need stems from physiological signals that the body sends out, nudging us to eat.[2] Some of these physiological signals are stomach growls and pains, weakness, headache, dizziness, anxiety, grumpiness (commonly known as being "hangry," which means being hungry and angry at the same time), difficulty concentrating, cravings, thirst, and a watering mouth.[3] Other than anxiety and being hangry, these signals are primarily physical, not emotional. These are the signals that indicate hunger, and they are often quite loud.

Now, what happens when you overlook these signals? As we discussed in the first section, when you restrict your food intake, your body interprets this action as a sign of impending danger. Your body recognizes that its **hunger signals** are not prompting you to nourish the body, so it switches gears. The body adapts to this perceived increased threat level and activates its survival instincts, transitioning to energy conservation mode.

As a result, the body diminishes the strength and frequency of these hunger signals while also slowing down thermogenesis to preserve its resources. It is an incredible example of how your body is wired to protect you, even when you might not realize you need protection.[4] In other words, even though you no longer feel as hungry as before, your body continues to go deeper into starvation mode, which is defined by a lack of nutrients and energy. People who continuously deprive themselves may develop anorexia nervosa.

Satiation

Now let us shift our focus to the concept of **satiation**. Feeling satiated, full, or satisfied, from a physiological standpoint, signifies that you are no longer in a state of hunger—your body is no longer craving nutrition—yet your stomach is not overly stuffed. Put simply, you have eaten just enough to pacify your body's hunger signals. The allure of food seems to fade, and you experience a sense of general well-being, as all the physiological cues associated with hunger have now subsided. It is that perfectly contented state where you have nourished your body just right.[5] It is important to note that it takes about twenty minutes for your body to register the presence of food in your stomach.

When you fail to heed the cues signaling that your body is no longer hungry, something else happens. This often occurs when you eat beyond the point of satisfaction, eat too quickly, or eat without mindfulness and don't allow your body to register the presence of food in your stomach. The result? You experience a feeling of pressure in your belly and start to feel unwell—stuffed to the brim, so to speak. You might experience some discomfort while breathing or moving, and you may even feel fatigued or need a nap.

As a child, you were naturally in sync with your body's cues. You ate when you felt hungry and stopped once the hunger faded. You felt content but not excessively full. It was as simple as that.

Where did we all go wrong? It happened when you started tuning in to cues and messages from outside your body and began adopting and emulating certain eating habits. You gradually drifted away from your instincts, and your eating style deviated from its natural state. In chapter 2, we discussed some of these influences:

- Listening to your parents telling you to finish everything on your plate
- Sitting down for dinner and eating everything that was served to you, whether you were that hungry or not
- Watching your parents dieting and telling you about good and bad food, instilling their diet mentality in you
- Seeing your parents, siblings, or friends eating and mimicking their consumption patterns

The result is that you stopped listening to yourself. To move further along your journey, you need to relearn your hunger and fullness cues and begin to pay attention to your body again.

In the next section, we focus on how you can permanently deprogram yourself from Diet Culture by understanding your body's cues. We will also explore the differences between emotional and situational reasons to eat versus our physical reasons to eat.

Section 2: Stopping Emotional and Mindless Eating

Let us see how Ava learned to discern between true hunger and fullness versus emotional or mindless eating.

Ava began to listen intently to her body's signals, learning to identify the distinct sensations of physical hunger—a rumbling stomach, lightheadedness, and a lack of energy—and understand them as her body's direct requests for nourishment. On the flip side, Ava also came face-to-face with emotional hunger, which was far less about her physical needs and more about her feelings. She recognized that emotional hunger would often manifest suddenly, triggered by stress, sadness, or even boredom, and it craved specific comfort foods rather than a well-rounded meal. It took practice, but Ava gradually mastered the art of distinguishing between the two types of hunger. She began to meet her emotional needs with self-care practices and responded to her physical hunger with nourishing meals that she ate mindfully. This newfound awareness not only improved her relationship with food but also enriched her overall well-being.

In this section, we are going to learn about emotional eating and mindless eating. Once we do that, we can begin to understand how they differ from eating to satisfy physical needs.

Mindless Eating

Mindless eating refers to consuming food in an environment riddled with distractions, when we lack any genuine awareness of or attention toward what we are eating. Remember, when we allow ourselves to be distracted during meals, we often lose sight of the body's natural hunger and satiety cues because our minds are preoccupied. Consequently, we may end up eating even when we are not hungry or when we surpass our natural satiety cues. Either path can lead to self-esteem issues, weight management challenges, or health concerns.

> When we allow ourselves to be distracted during meals, we often lose sight of the body's natural hunger and satiety cues because our minds are preoccupied.

Emotional Eating

On the other hand, emotional eating is influenced by specific emotional states, typically negative ones. As we saw with Ava, comfort eating is a prime example—this occurs when we are feeling anxious or down, and we tend to resort to high-fat, high-carb foods to create a semblance of warmth and nostalgia. Negative emotions often trigger binge eating, but it is important to note that emotional eating can be linked to positive emotions too, like the joyous feasting during holiday seasons. Regardless of whether emotional eating is driven by a positive or negative emotional state, the key characteristics involve consuming food when we are not hungry and often not stopping until we have surpassed satisfaction. It becomes a point of concern when someone consistently eats beyond the feeling of fullness.

Hunger and Fullness versus Emotional and Mindless Eating Exercise

In chapter 2, we discussed noticing the state of mind we were in during a day's meals to determine whether we were eating in an emotional or distracted state. Such introspection helps us identify the instances when we engage in these behaviors. We can now take this introspection to another level.

In this exercise, you will record what you eat to find out whether you have an awareness of the physical and emotional cues prompting you to eat. I would like you to track your eating habits, meals, and snacks for three days to get a clear picture of your regular eating habits—whether you are eating because of physical hunger or emotional reasons and how often you are eating for these reasons. Here are the steps you should complete for each meal of your day:

1. Record the time you eat.
2. Note your hunger level from 1–10, with 10 being the hungriest.
3. Evaluate your emotional state before eating.
4. Record your meal and the portion size of your meal. For example, a nine-inch bowl of Bolognese pasta with a slice of garlic bread.
5. List your meal setting, such as at the dinner table, in front of the television, at your desk at work, etc.
6. Note the percentage of the meal you ate. If you ate it all, note 100%.
7. Evaluate your emotional state after eating.
8. Record the time it took you to finish your meal.
9. Note your fullness level after eating, with 10 being the fullest.

> This exercise will help you figure out how often you eat when you are actually hungry, as opposed to when you are in some kind of emotional state, negative or positive. It also identifies how many of your meals are eaten in a distracted state and how fast you generally eat. You will also be able to identify whether you are listening to your fullness cues or eating well past fullness.

Once you have an idea of how much you eat when you are actually hungry and how much you eat when you are emotional or distracted, you can learn how to change your eating habits. You can begin listening to what your body needs and using its physical cues to help meet your goals.

Gaining awareness into the reasons you eat is key to relearning how to eat because of physiological hunger and when to stop once you feel satiated. You can practice this by simply tuning in to your body to search for physical signs of hunger as well as asking yourself what emotional state you are in.

Next, we will examine emotional cravings, how they are related to ignoring hunger and fullness, and how to change this to create better eating habits.

Section 3: Understanding Unhealthy Cravings

Let us see how Ava worked on her food cravings.

Before Ava began seeing me for therapy, she found herself caught in the challenging cycle of restrictive dieting. Aiming for a leaner physique, she willingly submitted herself to the stringent rules of a new diet, cutting out an entire spectrum of foods she once enjoyed. As time passed, Ava noticed an unusual pattern: she started craving foods high in fat and carbohydrates. These cravings, powerful and persistent, were not a mere test of her willpower, but an intense longing for the foods her diet had labeled as off limits.

Ava was taken aback by her body's vehement response to the lack of her beloved pasta and cheeseburgers. She began to question the sustainability of her restrictive diet, especially since it was leading her to obsess over the very foods she was trying to avoid. Together, we introduced balance and moderation back into her meals, and she began to allow herself to enjoy the foods she loved while still maintaining a health-conscious lifestyle. This shift led to an enlightening realization: A life of deprivation was not necessary for maintaining good health. Her cravings subsided, and she discovered a newfound, healthier relationship with food—one where no foods were labeled bad, and where balanced choices were readily available to her.

We are going to finish this chapter by examining how physical regulation works and how it can lead to food cravings when it does not work. It is important to establish this foundation before we explore practical ways to return to the more natural style of eating when hungry and stopping when satisfied. We'll delve into digestion to understand what happens in the body when we eat and how this relates to cravings. The body is regulated by many different hormones; we will focus on the two primary hormones involved in eating and digestion and learn how dieting can disrupt their functions and lead to food cravings.

Ghrelin

Ghrelin is a hormone made in and released primarily from the stomach, and like the "ghr" in its name, it is known as a hunger-producing hormone. Ghrelin makes us hungry, stimulates our appetites, controls insulin release, and increases the storage of fat. Ghrelin levels rise before we eat and lower after we eat, and the hormone is involved in the physical feelings of hunger.[6]

Ghrelin is the body's natural way to maintain balance. When we have excess weight, ghrelin levels decrease. When we fast or diet, or suffer from anorexia nervosa, ghrelin levels increase. Ghrelin increase during dieting plays a big role in increased food cravings because the body is pushing back, trying to return to a balance and maintain its weight.[7]

To put it simply, being mindful of your body's signals is crucial when you decide to make any lifestyle change. Setting a goal (like losing weight) does not magically translate into results. You need to lay out a path to guide your body along this journey that involves being in harmony with your body.

> Being mindful of your body's signals is crucial when you decide to make any lifestyle change.

Dieting often involves suppressing the appetite. This amplifies the production of ghrelin. Unfortunately, this makes us even hungrier and ramps up the odds of a binge-eating episode. So when your food cravings are persistent, they are essentially reaffirming a truth you have already heard: Dieting, in the traditional sense, falls short. If you tune in to your body, listen to your hunger signals, honor your cravings responsibly, and stop eating when full, you can maintain normal ghrelin levels.

Leptin

Leptin is a hormone released from fat cells that helps us regulate our food intake over time. In individuals considered to have a healthy weight, leptin works to stop fat deposition by regulating feeding behavior and energy balance and helps us survive periods of food deprivation.[8] In short, leptin tells you when you are no longer hungry.

When we lose weight, leptin levels fall. And when we lose weight aggressively, we trigger an automatic physical reaction from the body to correct for the drop in leptin. The result is a spike in appetite and food cravings, which are the body's way of telling us to increase fat production and storage to return to a balance.

When a person has excess weight, their body has higher levels of leptin. After some time at the increased weight, their body loses its sensitivity to leptin. This lack of sensitivity is like how we tune out the sound from a running fan in the background. A person will continue eating despite having sufficient fat storage, and despite having leptin levels signaling that they are no longer hungry. This results in weight gain.[9]

> By tuning in to your body when you are hungry and eating to the point of physical satisfaction, not overfullness, you can maintain steadier leptin levels, which will help you maintain a healthy, natural weight.

When you diet and consequently lose weight, your leptin levels dip, sparking cravings for high-calorie foods to counterbalance the fall. If you gain excessive weight, your body becomes somewhat immune to the high leptin levels, leading you to continue eating. By tuning in to your body when you are hungry and eating to the point of physical satisfaction, not overfullness, you can maintain steadier leptin levels, which will help you maintain a healthy, natural weight.

The crux of this change lies in reconnecting with your body, getting in sync with your natural rhythms, and heeding your body's needs. Robust research corroborates the idea that simply paying attention to the body enhances self-regulation, a topic we delved into earlier in this chapter. This improved self-regulation helps you understand when your body is hungry and when it is sufficiently nourished.[10] You are tuning in to your body's natural rhythms and *paying attention* to what your body needs. This is what Ava learned.

A heightened awareness of your body can be an immense help in managing and comprehending your physical cravings. It is time you started trusting your body again; it is innately programmed to desire food that boosts functionality. Essentially, when you are in tune with your body, you naturally gravitate toward healthy, nutrient-rich foods.

It is critical to be aware of an important point. You may desire foods of lower nutritional value when distracted or emotional, but these cravings do not align with your body's physical nutritional needs. As you become more mindful of your body, you are likely to choose healthier, more natural foods because these nourish your body best and keep you energized for extended periods between meals.[11]

> It is time you started trusting your body again; it is innately programmed to desire food that boosts functionality.

Like Ava, I trust you have gained insight into your hunger and fullness signals. I hope you are once again noticing these cues and have started distinguishing them from emotional and mindless eating. You may have also recognized that when you disregard these cues, your body will trigger cravings to restore balance or homeostasis. When you are attentive and self-regulate, your body will nudge you to fuel it with nutrient-dense foods like veggies, whole grains, lean proteins, and healthy fats. Essentially, your body will ask for the foods that will help you operate at your best, physically and mentally—not only like a finely tuned Ferrari, but one with a sharp and skilled driver at the wheel!

In the next chapter, we will confront thoughts that are no longer beneficial to us. We must shake off old, entrenched negative thinking patterns that have, both metaphorically and literally, held us back and weighed us down. This transformation will guide us on a journey toward a healthier, more natural life—a life where we can enjoy any food we want, whenever we please!

Chapter 4

YOU ARE YOUR OWN WORST ENEMY—HOW TO BE YOUR BEST FRIEND

Introduction

This chapter will examine how your thoughts can be your worst enemies. We will focus on three fundamental objectives:

- Identifying negative and unhelpful thoughts
- Identifying better, kinder, and more helpful thoughts
- Changing your thoughts for good

By the end of this chapter, you will know how to become more self-compassionate, how to be a better friend to yourself, and how to achieve greater happiness and better health.

Section 1: Examine Your Thoughts

Ezra had been adopted by a family at a young age. Unfortunately, his adoptive mother was constantly critical of him and his behavior. This constant criticism caused the young boy to strive for perfection in every aspect of his life. He wanted to make his adoptive mother proud and show her that he was worth the efforts she put into raising him. Ezra was an excellent student and a talented athlete. He worked hard in school and in his extracurricular activities to make sure he was succeeding. He was successful in most areas of his life, but the constant criticism from his adoptive mother made him doubt himself and his accomplishments.

Ezra's constant need to be perfect eventually led him down a dangerous path as an adult. He believed that if he was not perfect in every way, he would never be accepted. He started to binge eat when he felt out of control and then would starve himself to regain control over his life. Ezra's issue had a serious impact on his health. He was always exhausted, and his work began to suffer. He was constantly in emotional pain and unable to concentrate on work or his social life. Eventually, he came to me for treatment.

In this chapter, we will examine how your thoughts, like Ezra's, can work against you, especially when it comes to body image. To truly appreciate this influence, we need to understand a little bit of psychological theory—specifically, Cognitive Behavioral Therapy.

Cognitive Behavioral Therapy (CBT)

Back in the 1960s, a visionary named Aaron T. Beck introduced the world to **Cognitive Behavioral Therapy (CBT)**. This therapeutic approach has been instrumental in helping people navigate through a myriad of mental disorders, from depression and anxiety to eating disorders and obsessive-compulsive disorder. Central to CBT is the profound connection between thoughts, feelings, and behaviors.

Here is a relatable example. Let us say you have a thought like this: "The world is unsafe." This thought might trigger feelings of anxiety or panic. These feelings could then provoke physical reactions such as hyperventilation, tension, insomnia, or a full-blown panic attack.

This is where CBT shines. It equips you with the tools to transform those disruptive thoughts into something more constructive and positive. Take the earlier thought, for example, and imagine changing it to this: "I am safe right now." Such a shift can help you cultivate a sense of calmness and give you space to pause, take some deep and soothing breaths, and better manage your reactions.[1]

How does CBT apply to your thoughts about food and eating? Over time, you may have developed some negative thinking patterns about food and eating, such as the following:

- Maladaptive schemas
- Cognitive distortions
- Repetitive negative thinking (rumination)

I'll explain each of these patterns because one of the most important steps in your journey is identifying when these occur. They may appear independently or together.

Maladaptive Schemas

Beck defined a **maladaptive schema** as a long-standing, long-lasting, dysfunctional or self-defeating pattern of thinking developed in childhood or adolescence that informs a negative belief about the self, the world, or the future. These schemas produce negative automatic thoughts, especially with regard to weight and shape.[2]

Cognitive Distortions

Cognitive distortions are essentially exaggerated or skewed views of reality that can profoundly influence your relationship with food. These distortions can take several forms. You might find yourself taking things personally, interpreting every situation as a direct reflection of how people feel about you. Or perhaps you are prone to catastrophic thinking, where you envision the worst possible outcome for every circumstance. It is also possible that you perceive the world in absolutes, sorting everything into good versus bad, or black-and-white buckets.[3]

Fascinating research has shed light on the power of cognitive distortions and their impact on eating behaviors. For instance, it is common for people to equate consuming high-calorie foods with immediate feelings of becoming fatter; people believe they have instantly gained weight or think they have made a moral transgression. This type of distorted thinking was found to be more common among individuals considered to have normal weight than those who were considered overweight. It just goes to show how our mindsets can greatly affect our behaviors, including those related to food.[4]

Repetitive Negative Thinking (Rumination)

Repetitive negative thinking, also called rumination, is an extreme fixation by the individual on the negative thought to the point that it colors their perception, influences their choices, and is constantly a focal point in their conversations. Rumination has been linked to a higher prevalence of disordered behavior. Specifically, repetitive negative thinking caused people to weigh themselves repeatedly and check the body parts they did not like in the mirror more often.[5]

These are just some examples of the types of thinking that can cause you to view yourself and your body in a negative light, generate misconceptions about food, and lead you to believe you are unworthy. Ezra strove for perfection to obtain his mother's approval, but those thinking patterns caused unhealthy binging and restricting behaviors. Similarly, negative thinking patterns can leave you feeling terrible about yourself—guilty, shameful, undeserving, and unloved. Such emotions can, in turn, push you toward excessive dieting, obsessive weight-checking, and constant scrutiny of your body's perceived imperfections.

It is important to acknowledge that these thought patterns are common. Rarely does anyone navigate through our toxic diet-centric society without picking up a few of these distortions or negative beliefs. The fact that these thought patterns are universal, however, means we all must overcome them on the journey to healthier self-perception.

To develop healthier thought patterns, it helps to identify your most deeply held negative thoughts about yourself and your food. This helps you become aware of your negative schemas, cognitive distortions, and recurring negative thoughts. Take a moment to think about the answer(s) to this question: Which negative schemas, cognitive distortions, or recurring negative thoughts do you find yourself wrestling with? By identifying these patterns, you can start to make changes to improve your mental, physical, and emotional well-being.

> Rarely does anyone navigate through our toxic diet-centric society without picking up a few of these distortions or negative beliefs.

Sometimes, we can be our own harshest critics. Do you frequently check yourself in the mirror, weigh yourself, opt for oversized clothing, or perhaps avoid mirrors altogether? Do you shun carbs entirely? Push yourself to exercise until you are exhausted? Endlessly scroll through Instagram for "fitspiration"? If left unchecked, negative thoughts can lead to a cycle of misery, dieting, and self-loathing.

But what if you started to be nicer to yourself? What if you became your own cheerleader? How might you change your internal dialogue to accomplish that?

You can develop a new approach to thinking, feeling, and behaving. You can create helpful changes by altering the fundamentals of your thought processes. Picture a world where your thoughts about yourself are only positive. What if you could let go of the constant self-scrutiny and body checking? Does this sound far-fetched?

It is possible. I remind my clients, "You are not your thoughts." Just because you have thought a certain way for a long time does not mean that is the core of who you are. Changing your thoughts can change your life.

I hope this sheds some light on your thought processes and how they can limit you. If left unchecked, your thoughts can be your own worst enemy. But becoming aware of these thoughts is just the beginning. In the next section, we will explore ways to reshape our thinking. We will see the profound impact this shift can have on your life, your eating patterns, your breathing, and your capacity to love yourself.

> Changing your thoughts can change your life.

Section 2: Change Your Thoughts

Before Ezra became my client, his pursuit of an ideal physique had begun to take a toll on his body and mental health. He adopted extreme dietary restrictions and relentless exercise routines. He meticulously counted every calorie and shied away from any food he deemed unhealthy. Despite these restrictions, Ezra would find himself periodically succumbing to uncontrollable binges—raiding the fridge late at night and consuming everything he had denied himself during the day. This left him feeling guilt-ridden and trapped in a vicious cycle of restriction and overeating. Ezra was perplexed, unable to understand why his pursuit of perfection was leading him down such a tumultuous path.

It was not until I introduced him to the idea of cognitive distortions that Ezra began to comprehend the root of his struggle. He recognized his pursuit of perfection as a form of all-or-nothing thinking, a cognitive distortion where he was classifying his actions, especially concerning diet and exercise, as "perfect" or "failure.'"

This understanding was a revelation. Ezra realized that his distorted thoughts were driving his unhealthy relationship with food. His rigid dietary restrictions were born out of a fear of failing to maintain the perfect diet. And when he inevitably and understandably slipped, he would end up binge eating, fueled by feelings of guilt and failure. This revelation allowed us to begin to examine and—most importantly—change these thoughts.

In the last section, we embarked on an introspective journey, examining the thoughts that might be diminishing your joy and holding you firmly in the clutches of Diet Culture. Now, we will dive into the exciting task of transforming these unhelpful perceptions for the better. Remember, patience is paramount. These thoughts did not appear overnight; they are the result of a lifetime's worth of experiences, so they will require some effort to reshape.

Thus far, we have highlighted the negative impacts on your goals that can be caused by negative thoughts about your body and your eating habits. In this chapter, we will see that you have the power to rewire these harmful thinking patterns. Do not despair. It does not take another lifetime to undo the damage. What it does take is consistency and regular practice.

Extensive research confirms the effectiveness of CBT as a reliable and safe treatment for the behaviors and core symptoms associated with eating disorders. CBT focuses on the thoughts that trigger feelings of distress that lead to negative behaviors. When we break down our thinking, we often realize that our negative thoughts lack substantial evidence and, surprisingly, we often find more proof supporting the contrary interpretation.[6] Once we acknowledge that our thinking may be unduly leaning toward negativity, it is like a breath of fresh air lightening our mental load and clearing the way for a shift in our thought patterns. When we purposefully analyze our thoughts, particularly those focused on our weight, body shape, and beliefs about food, we empower ourselves to alter them and thus enhance our overall thinking, emotional well-being, and functioning.

> But when a negative thought has dominated our mental landscape for years, the evidence against it tends to get overlooked because our attention is predominantly drawn toward the negative. That is why shifting our focus can be transformative.

Throughout my practice as a psychologist and dietitian, I have interacted with numerous clients who questioned their self-worth. Many have carried the intensely negative yet surprisingly common belief that they are worthless. My approach involves challenging these ingrained beliefs, asking clients to gather any evidence that supports their feelings of worthlessness—any instances of others confirming or treating them as such. I then guide them through a process in which they contrast this negativity with evidence that they are worthwhile and loved.

I urge them to recall moments when someone expressed love or gratitude for their friendship. Almost invariably, everyone can remember many instances where they have been valued and appreciated. But when a negative thought has dominated our mental landscape for years, the evidence against it tends to get overlooked because our attention is predominantly drawn toward the negative. That is why shifting our focus can be transformative.

What if the evidence refuting these negative thoughts is, in fact, overwhelming? Together, we can set out to shape a new, healthier thought. What if, instead of constantly thinking, "I am worthless," you began to believe, "I am a compassionate and loving friend, deserving of time and attention." Ponder the emotional impact of such a change in thought.

Imagine how it feels to reflect on instances where you have been a wonderful friend to a loved one. What emotions surface? Perhaps joy, pride, a sense of being loved, or gratitude? Time and again, my clients report a heartening warmth and satisfaction when they revisit these memories. As they summon these heartwarming memories, they have a breakthrough moment when they realize that they are the source of these uplifting feelings. This is the kind of thought restructuring I did with Ezra. If you can cultivate healthier thoughts and consequently more positive feelings, how might this influence your behavior? Let us explore that further.

When individuals start to embrace the positive feelings kindled by their own memories, it generates an enhanced sense of self-worth, leading to an increased sense of joy and the feeling of being loved. This emotional uplift encourages further self-kindness, greater empathy toward others, and increased involvement in positive activities. Through this transformative process, you can reshape your thoughts and ultimately improve your self-perception. But remember, practice and patience are required. After all, if you have spent a significant portion of your life entertaining negative thoughts about yourself, it is going to take some time to develop the habit of thinking positively.

How can you translate this idea to your attitudes about food? Suppose your prevailing thought is "All carbs are bad." How does that influence your feelings? Perhaps it triggers a sense of guilt when you consume carbs or self-reproach when you deviate from your carb-free regimen. Consequently, how do you behave? You might avoid carbs like the plague, only to eventually give in, binge on carb-rich food like mac-n-cheese, and then resort to a drastic measure like a five-day juice cleanse as a form of self-punishment. What a brutal cycle of self-loathing and torment!

Why do we say that all carbs are bad? Even though certain types of carbs are metabolized into glucose more rapidly than others (for example, a doughnut versus a piece of whole-grain bread), carbs in their various forms are essential for our survival. The body needs glucose for optimal brain function, for energy, and for regulating our cholesterol levels. Carbohydrates, therefore, are essential to our health. This becomes our evidence against the harmful belief, "All carbs are bad." How about shifting this thought to "We need carbs"?

When you adopt this healthier perspective, how does your behavior change? You cease demonizing an entire food group and remove the taboo status associated with it. Carbohydrates become an essential part of your dietary choices instead of a forbidden temptation. It might be challenging to shake off the deeply ingrained notion perpetuated by Diet Culture that carbs are bad, but the new perspective I am proposing can liberate you from the cycle of restriction and starvation and the ensuing guilt and shame when you do consume them. This shift in thought greatly helped Ezra reformulate his relationship with food.

You can ensure these fresh perspectives take root by cultivating awareness. By consciously recognizing these thoughts as they surface, rather than letting them slip into your mind unnoticed, you are empowered to disrupt the cycle of detrimental, counterproductive thinking. These are the insights Ezra began to develop.

> It might be challenging to shake off the deeply ingrained notion perpetuated by Diet Culture that carbs are bad, but the new perspective I am proposing can liberate you from the cycle of restriction and starvation and the ensuing guilt and shame when you do consume them.

The goal is to identify these thoughts as they arise, then consciously recall your healthier alternatives and thereby reshape your mindset for the long term. This is the technique you will be practicing in the upcoming section. For now, I hope you realize that a wealth of evidence contradicts your old negative thought patterns. You are now equipped to replace these with kinder, more self-compassionate thoughts. In our next section, we will delve into how to put this fresh way of thinking into practice!

Section 3: Practice Makes Perfect

Recognizing distorted thoughts was Ezra's first step toward change. He decided to replace his pursuit of perfection with the goal of balance and self-compassion. Instead of restricting certain foods, Ezra began to embrace all foods, focusing on nutrition and how they made his body feel. When he felt the urge to binge, he would pause and remind himself that it was his body's natural response to restriction and not a personal failure. He also reminded himself that occasional indulgences are a normal part of a balanced diet and do not equate to failing.

Ezra's journey is far from over. There are still days when the old thoughts creep back in, but he now has the tools to recognize and challenge these cognitive distortions. His story serves as a reminder that perfection is an illusion and that the pursuit of balance, self-compassion, and mindfulness can pave the way for a healthier relationship with food.

In the previous section, we explored ways to shift your thoughts from negative and counterproductive to more compassionate and constructive. But is it as simple as it sounds? Can you just decide on a new way of thinking and—voilà—you are transformed for good?

I would love to assure you that modifying your thought patterns is an effortless process, but the truth is, it is not easy. The concept is straightforward, but putting it into practice requires effort. Yet, with consistent practice, a new pattern is absolutely achievable!

> The pursuit of balance, self-compassion,
> and mindfulness can pave the way for
> a healthier relationship with food.

In this section, we will explore how to practice your newfound thoughts in dynamic, engaging, and creative ways. Practice may make perfect, but it certainly does not have to be monotonous or tedious. We are going to kick things off with a technique called Thought Stopping.

Thought Stopping

Thought Stopping is a strategy derived from CBT and is designed to help individuals curb their negative thoughts. When originally applied within a therapy session, the client ponders troubling thoughts. The therapist abruptly exclaims, "Stop!" Subsequently, the client articulates their thoughts and then says aloud, "Stop!" Finally, the client silently says, "Stop!" when those thoughts emerge.

This technique has proven effective in addressing a wide array of issues, ranging from anxiety and depression to obsessive-compulsive disorder and eating disorders. When coupled with positive techniques and self-talk, Thought Stopping serves as a potent coping mechanism, aiding in the cessation of negative thought patterns and rumination.[7] You will use a variant of Thought Stopping combined with the repetitive use of mantras to steadily shift your thoughts in a more positive direction. Now, you might be thinking,

"Mantras? That sounds a bit mystical!" It might seem mystical, but we will demystify it together!

Mantras

Mantras, in essence, are words or phrases that are continuously repeated during meditation. Repeating a mantra helps any other internal or external distractions gently fade into the background. The purpose of repeating the selected word or phrase is to trigger a state of relaxation. Although it may sound mystical, it is intended to help us cultivate tranquility and focus.[8]

Mantras might seem a bit odd due to their portrayal in popular culture—like the classic "Om" chanting in Transcendental Meditation, images of individuals sitting serenely in lotus position atop mountains, or people participating in rejuvenating sound baths. It may seem a tad "out there," but I believe that is because repeating mantras is unfamiliar to most people. Having said that, I would wager that many of you have actually been practicing your own mantras more often than you realize!

Have you ever found yourself repeating phrases like "I can do it!" or "I got this!" in your head or out loud? Those affirmations, when repeated, function as mantras and can be particularly powerful when combined with relaxation techniques.

I often introduce mantra meditation to my clients who are navigating the challenges of deprogramming from Diet Culture. This technique is a superb tool for enhancing positive mental health, alleviating negative moods, reducing stress, and promoting a clearer and more focused mind. The "woo-woo" veneer is simply a matter of unfamiliarity, but mantra meditation is a practical and potent tool for personal transformation.[9] This powerful form of meditation can serve as an effective tool to help you reshape your thoughts. It is quite common for my clients to start crafting their own mantras during our sessions, having recognized their potential to combat negative thinking.

I help my clients use mantras to effectively transition from negative thoughts to positive actions. We start by having them identify their most negative self-perceptions and beliefs about food. From there, we work together to craft a mantra that directly challenges these thoughts with facts. And then I help them practice these personalized mantras. Many of my clients have found this process to be remarkably transformative.

Create Your Own Mantra

The following is a condensed version of the process for creating your own mantra. Let us say you are struggling to shake the message that carbs are bad, and you find it influencing you while grocery shopping or ordering at a restaurant. The first step is to directly challenge this thought with a fact. You know that carbs are vital for your brain and body functions. From there, you can create a short mantra to remind yourself of this fact, such as "My body needs carbs," or "Carbs are healthy." If you fear that eating a single brownie will cause weight gain, you could counteract this by remembering what you have learned so far in this book. You can say, "I can enjoy food more if I listen to my body," or "I eat when I am hungry, and I will stop when I am full." One of Ezra's new mantras is "I listen to my body," and it works amazingly well for him.

Coupling mantras with Thought Stopping can really set your new thoughts in motion. This is when your awareness comes into play. It is essential to start observing your thoughts on a moment-to-moment basis. This might sound challenging because we often operate on autopilot and are not tuned in to our internal dialogue. But with this newfound understanding of your thoughts, you will be equipped to notice them as they occur.

Certain people or situations often trigger these negative thoughts. Perhaps you chat with an overly critical colleague or a gossipy friend who leaves you feeling insignificant. It is easy to spiral into self-doubt, perhaps turning to comfort food like a doughnut to soothe the sting. This is the moment to pause. Say "stop" to yourself, find a quiet spot, close your eyes, and steady your breath. Acknowledge that you are feeling bad about yourself, breathe in and out slowly, become aware of the negative thought that is surfacing, and replace it with your newly formed mantra.

Bring your mantra to your conscious mind. If it is "I am loved," then repeat this phrase to yourself as many times as necessary until you feel a sense of calm washing over you. After five minutes of quiet breathing and mantra repetition, you might discover you are less anxious, feel safer, and experience a stronger sense of love. And guess what? You may not even crave that doughnut anymore. You will likely feel calm, comforted, and at peace.

I urge all my clients to try this coping technique at least three times, and I hope you will do the same. You might start noticing its benefits straight away, but bear in mind, new behaviors take time and practice to become habits. As the saying goes, practice makes perfect. Once you realize how good you feel, you will naturally be motivated to make this a habit.

Later in this book we will dive deeper into the concept of habits. But for now, you are laying the groundwork for healthier habits by reshaping your thoughts. This change requires consistent reminders for practice, and I have a fun, creative way to achieve this.

Post-it Notes

How will you remember to use your new mantra? It is simple—you will use Post-it notes! Are they not fantastic? You can stick them practically anywhere as a handy visual reminder of your new mantra. I suggest you write down your mantra and place the notes in areas that might trigger negative thoughts, such as your bathroom mirror, your desk, near the TV, on the fridge, or even at your workplace.

If you are worried about others seeing the notes and poking fun, you can always use a unique symbol that represents your mantra. Whatever symbol or image you choose, ensure it triggers the memory of your mantra and evokes a positive emotion. And remember, while you may not always be able to avoid certain people, like that gossip in the office, you can keep your mantra safe by having your unique symbol. If you find that the people closest to you belittle this practice, perhaps you might reconsider the amount of time you spend with them.

Throughout this process, it is crucial to surround yourself with supportive, loving individuals who encourage your growth. Anyone who mocks this process might need to reflect on their own negative thoughts. Show compassion for them, but also make sure to prioritize your own well-being.

I hope this section has armed you with practical and productive tools for change. By consistently using mantras, you can establish healthier, more compassionate, and empathetic thought patterns. You are well on your way to becoming healthier, just like Ezra! Remember, putting what you have learned into practice will greatly assist you as you move forward. Brace yourself for a fresh, more enjoyable perspective on eating and living.

Chapter 5

THE PRESENT MOMENT IS A GIFT

Introduction

In this chapter, you will learn how mindfulness and the art of mindful eating can help you deprogram yourself out of Diet Culture and reintroduce yourself to the love and joy of eating. We discuss three fundamental topics:

- How mindfulness can help you on your journey
- How mindful eating can help you self-regulate to maintain a healthy weight
- How to practice mindful eating during your meals

Section 1: What Is Mindfulness?

Grace, a vibrant woman with an infectious smile, had an intriguing story that began in her childhood. As a child, she was short and round, a size and shape that displeased her parents. They often commented on this, comparing her to her taller, thinner sister. Grace, a tender soul, carried the painful stings of their hurtful comments deep within her.

These experiences started a cycle where Grace began to dissociate during meals. It was as though she was floating outside of herself, observing a girl who mechanically consumed her food without tasting or enjoying it. Eating became a solitary act, devoid of pleasure or satisfaction, serving only to fuel her body.

Despite her best efforts to shield herself with well-planned outfits, Grace constantly felt like an imposter. The woman who stared back at her from the mirror did not match the vibrant, confident individual she presented to the world. A silent, uneasy question lingered in her heart: "Would they still accept me if they saw the real Grace?"

Over time, Grace realized that these protective strategies, while serving a purpose in the past, were no longer beneficial. In fact, they were barriers, preventing her from truly embracing and loving herself. She decided it was time to reawaken and rewrite her narrative, to move from feeling like an imposter to becoming an authentic version of herself. That is when she came to see me.

I worked with Grace to help her develop mindful eating habits. **Mindfulness** is being aware of the present moment and accepting it in a nonjudgmental, open-hearted manner.[1] It is based on Eastern Buddhist traditions such as Theravada Buddhism and Zen Buddhism, and it was first made popular in the United States and Europe by Jon Kabat-Zinn as a stress-reduction treatment for chronic pain.[2] This mindfulness-based stress-reduction treatment was then combined with CBT to form **Mindfulness-Based Cognitive Therapy** (MBCT); applying this technique has improved many different types of mental illnesses: depression, anxiety, obsessive-compulsive disorder, eating disorders, and more. MBCT attempts to change depressive ruminative thinking about the past or anxiety regarding the future by switching from the "doing mind" to the "being mind."[3]

First, I will explain the concept of the "doing mind."

> Mindfulness is being aware of the present moment and accepting it in a nonjudgmental, open-hearted manner.

The Doing Mind

Becoming fully present is not only about a conscious decision to do so; it also involves letting go of the subconscious filters that tint your perception. Those subconscious filters are what constitute the "doing mind." They keep you from simply meeting the world as it is, without judgment.

Take observing your surroundings, for example. You may be including subjective judgments with your observations. Imagine a woman strolling down the street. Instead of simply observing the objective facts, such as the color of her attire, are you also categorizing her according to societal norms—labeling her as thin or curvy, beautiful or ordinary, alluring or not? Are you defining her based on preconceived ideas about what a woman should resemble?

You might be thinking, "Well, what is the harm in that?" Inherently, these comparisons are brimming with judgment, which often leads us to classify things as good or bad, positive or negative. And, as we have previously explored with food, this binary thinking can lead us to demonize certain foods. Let us imagine for a moment that we stripped away those judgments.

What if food was just food—neither good nor bad, just simply food? What if you refrained from comparing people to each other or yourself, and instead of labeling them, you just saw them as individuals, without any feelings of competition, aspiration, or envy? This is the thought process you can foster through mindfulness. This is the new thought process that Grace began to adopt.

The Being Mind

> Being fully present means being aware of and accepting the current moment in a nonjudgmental, open-hearted way.

The "being mind" is a mindset rooted in the present moment without any comparative references or judgments. How do we shift from a "doing mind" to a "being mind"? The key lies in the definition: Being fully present means being aware of and accepting the current moment in a nonjudgmental, openhearted way. Awareness is the key point here.

If you recall what you learned in the previous chapters, you will see that you have been cultivating self-awareness all along—you have been practicing mindfulness this whole time! You have worked on reframing many of your thoughts about yourself and your relationship with food, promoting kindness and compassion. You have been breaking free from mindless and emotional eating and learning to tune in to your body. And you have been doing all of this through increased awareness. Now, we are about to take this practice a step further.

We are going to explore how to stay present in each moment, approaching it with an open heart and without judgment. Mindfulness exercises help alleviate feelings of depression and anxiety by **grounding** you in the present, enabling you to tune in to your surroundings without judgment or criticism. The beauty of mindfulness exercises is their accessibility. A quiet, comfortable spot is all you need to bring yourself back to the present moment.

> **Mindfulness Grounding Exercise**
>
> Either read from the exercise below or visit our meditations web page to participate in this exercise by pointing your phone's camera at the QR code below and following the link to our Meditation Videos page at anew-insight.com.

continued

Before we embark on this exercise, take a moment to tune in to your emotions. What are you feeling right now? Perhaps you are a bit down or tired, or maybe you are experiencing a wave of joy?

Let's begin the exercise:

1. Start with the rhythm of your breath. Breathe in for a count of five and exhale for the same count. Inhale, exhale. Let your focus rest solely on your breath—inhale for five counts, then exhale for five counts. Do this for at least five breaths.
2. Next, engage your senses. Start with your sight. Take a gentle look around your room and merely observe. Without assigning any judgment, acknowledge what you see—a lamp, a table, a carpet, a window, or anything else that captures your attention.
3. Now, shift your awareness to your hearing. What sounds reach your ears? Maybe it is a ticking clock, the hum of the air conditioner, or the voices of people outside. Just notice these auditory elements around you.
4. Next, engage your sense of smell. Can you detect any particular odors? Perhaps a hint of perfume, a room deodorizer, or the comforting scent of fresh laundry? Simply make a mental note of the scents.
5. Now, focus on touch. What sensations can you feel around you? Is your seat firm or plush? What textures can your hands perceive?
6. Finally, explore taste. What flavors linger in your mouth? Have you just finished a meal or maybe brushed your teeth? Take a moment to notice your taste sensations.
7. Now, go back to your breath—inhale for five counts, then exhale for five counts. Do this for five more breaths.

> 8. To wrap up this exercise, bring your attention back to your feelings and emotions.
>
> Every person I have shared this exercise with has reported feeling more peaceful, serene, and anchored in the present moment afterward. This, my friends, is mindfulness. In my opinion, it is the gateway to happiness. Did you notice that the exercise does not dwell on any past events or future worries? You simply sat, observed, and allowed yourself to "be," rather than "do." This was a particularly mind-opening experience for Grace.

To conclude this section, I would like to share one of my all-time favorite quotes, which fittingly comes from the movie *Kung Fu Panda*. The wise old turtle, Oogway, imparts some valuable wisdom about emotional eating and mindfulness to Kung Fu Panda. He says, "Yesterday is history, tomorrow is a mystery, but today is a gift. That is why it is called the present."

That, in essence, is mindfulness encapsulated in a nutshell (or a turtle shell, if you prefer). It holds the key to happiness. And just like Master Oogway, now that you understand this sage wisdom, you are going to apply it to mindful eating.

Section 2: What Is Mindful Eating?

Let us see how Grace transformed her relationship with eating.

The journey was not easy, but Grace embraced the challenge. She learned to reframe her thoughts and replace the old, harmful beliefs with new, empowering ones. She explored techniques like mantra meditation, finding solace in phrases like "I am enough" and "I am beautiful just as I am."

Just as she transformed her relationship with herself, Grace began to transform her relationship with food, moving from dissociation to **mindful eating**. Through our work together, she rediscovered how to eat mindfully as she did when she was very young. By tapping into her senses and allowing herself to just be, Grace began to find joy in the sensory pleasure of eating. She learned to savor each bite and allow herself to experience the flavors, textures, and aromas of her meals. Eating slowly, she was now present in the moment, enjoying her food without guilt or the need to disconnect. Grace learned that mindful eating is a healthier and more natural approach to finding joy in her everyday meals.

In the late 1990s, researchers Jean Kristeller and C. Brendan Hallett found that many strategies used in Mindfulness-Based Cognitive Therapy (MBCT), originally devised for depression and anxiety, could be extended to address issues related to eating.[4] They developed what is known as **Mindfulness-Based Eating Awareness Training** to treat binge eating disorder. Their findings were promising—their approach led to a decrease in binge eating and incidences of depression while significantly enhancing the client's sense of control.

Their research shed light on the power of combining self-regulation and increased mindfulness. This duo was found to be effective in tackling oversensitivity to emotional, social, or behaviorally conditioned triggers, such as advertising and peer pressure. Moreover, it helped individuals tune in to their body's hunger and fullness cues.[5] In further research, they found that the *quantity* of mindfulness practice was a predictor of improvement in weight loss, and binge eating decreased in direct relationship to the *degree*, or more specifically the *amount*, of mindfulness practice.[6] In essence, their findings suggested that the more the individuals practiced mindfulness, the higher their chances of achieving their weight-loss goals and curbing their binge-eating tendencies. Fascinating, right?

Does the term "self-regulation" ring a bell? It came up in our discussion about distinguishing between hunger and fullness, as well as understanding emotional or mindless eating. As we learned in the previous chapter, mindfulness—experiencing the present moment fully—is the key to happiness, and self-regulation is crucial to understanding hunger and satiety cues.

> The more the individuals practiced mindfulness, the higher their chances of achieving their weight-loss goals and curbing their binge-eating tendencies.

Recall that mindfulness is an open-hearted, nonjudgmental awareness of the present moment. You can focus this same level of awareness on your food, without attaching labels of good or bad. Contrast this with the concept of mindless eating, which is the opposite of mindfulness. Mindless eating tends to happen when you are distracted—perhaps watching TV, scrolling on your computer, or socializing. The food in front of you is often overlooked or only partially acknowledged. Sometimes you may consume food so quickly that you barely get to savor it. Mindless, emotional eating can also occur—imagine rushing home after a stressful day and mindlessly eating a tub of ice cream in front of the TV, despite not being hungry enough to eat at all.

When you eat mindfully, you fully embrace the sensory experience of the food. You appreciate its delicious aroma and its tantalizing appearance. You acknowledge the shape, the colors, and the fragrance. You take the time to truly enjoy the first bite, letting the flavors play on the tongue. You notice the texture—is it crunchy, chewy, soft, or hard? You take pleasure in every mouthful, listening to your body as it signals satiety. The aim is not to overeat but to reach a point of satisfaction. Can you remember the last time you savored a meal in this way? Many of us cannot. But when you do, I assure you, overeating and overindulgence become things of the past. This approach can help you realize why no foods should be strictly off limits.

Mindful eating allows your body to guide you toward the foods you need. Over time, tuning in to your body will reveal that wholesome, nutritious foods filled with fiber, nutrients, and flavor help you function better. You might notice that after a few potato chips, your body signals, "All right, that is enough." You will understand that the cravings for salt- or sugar-laden treats only occur occasionally, and usually a few bites are all you desire. There are no forbidden foods—you are free to eat what you want, when you want. When you are truly in sync with your body, you eat when you are hungry and stop when you have had enough. This simple approach can help you maintain a healthy weight effortlessly.

Grace felt a great release when she learned to listen to her body and realized she could enjoy any food she desired, whenever she pleased. Grace discovered this was true freedom and joy. And I am sure you will experience the same joy if you try!

Section 3: Mindful Eating Practice

Grace began to see that eating mindfully was a joy and not a chore or something to be feared. She set out to incorporate this newfound knowledge as part of her routine. She learned a lengthier exercise from me (which is included in the online course) that helped her build a strong foundation of mindful eating, but she needed a way to be able to do this easily with every meal. She adopted some of the strategies found in this section, and mindful eating became a regular part of her daily life. Through her journey, Grace discovered that the only approval she needed was her own. The woman she now saw reflected back in the mirror was authentically her—vibrant, brave, and beautiful. Grace's story is a testament to her courage and resilience. It is a journey of self-discovery, self-awareness, self-acceptance, and most importantly, self-love. And the best part is that she continues to evolve and make gentle, transformative changes.

In this section, you will learn how to practice mindful eating and turn it into a new habit. As with any new practice, it takes a little bit of time to get used to doing something new.

Mindful Eating Mini-Exercise

This simplified version of a mindful eating exercise will help you practice awareness of your senses while eating. It will help you identify your hunger and mood, enhance your self-awareness, and refine your self-regulation. A more comprehensive version of this exercise can be found in my online course, if needed.

For this activity, I encourage you to eliminate any distractions other than calming music. Switch off your phone, computer, or tablet to fully focus on the experience.

1. Begin by taking a moment to sit comfortably and focus on your breathing. Take a deep breath in, then exhale. Repeat this and, while doing so, appreciate your surroundings.
2. Next, I would like you to rate your hunger level on a scale of 1 to 10, with 10 being extremely hungry. Ideally, your hunger level should be around 7 when you sit down to eat. A score lower than that might suggest you are not quite ready to eat. But remember to try not to allow your hunger to exceed 7, as that can often lead to faster eating and overeating.
3. Now, check in with your emotional state. Ask yourself what you are feeling. Are you angry, serene, content, melancholic, joyous, irritable, frustrated, playful, elated, anxious, despondent, or something else?
4. Next, take some time to observe your food. Notice the colors and the presentation.
5. Then, breathe in the aromas. Identify the different scents without forming any judgment—simply acknowledge them.
6. Listen to the ambient sounds around you. It could be some music, laughter, or the hum of your surroundings.
7. Next, explore your sense of touch. If you are eating with your hands, focus on the feel of your food. Or focus on the sensation of holding a fork, the napkin in your lap, or even the texture of the table and the seat cushion.
8. Now, take a bite of your food. Allow it to rest in your mouth for a moment before you chew. Experience the

continued

flavors, the texture, the delightful sensation of your meal. Savor each bite, indulging in the sensory feast.

9. After eating for about ten minutes, evaluate your satiety. Could you stop now and feel content? Or do you still feel physically hungry and crave more food? Ideally, a level of 7 on your fullness scale indicates satisfaction. A level of 9 or 10 indicates you have overeaten beyond your genuine hunger. If that happens, do not fret! It is all about practicing and getting better with time.

10. Finally, reassess your emotional state. You might feel content, relaxed, joyous, or peaceful.

When you fully engage in a mindful activity, you may lose track of time, becoming absorbed in the moment. This is what you should aim to achieve when eating mindfully. You should be fully immersed in the delightful sensory experience of eating, without self-criticism or comparisons.

By doing this, you will start to observe that nutritious foods—rich in fiber, vitamins, minerals, and vibrant colors—keep you energized for longer and make you feel your best. Less healthy options may not give you the same feeling, and you might find yourself gravitating toward healthier alternatives more frequently. But remember, the choice is always yours.

You will also realize that you can enjoy that piece of cake, but instead of finishing it off in one go (like you might have done before), you might feel satisfied with just a few bites, knowing you can always have more later if you wish. Doesn't that sound heavenly?

I hope this chapter has equipped you with the tools you need to incorporate mindfulness and mindful eating into your daily routine. With these tools, combined with what you have already learned, you are laying the groundwork for lifelong habits of self-love and food appreciation. This is what Grace learned. And like Grace, you can create a life free from the negative cycle of dieting, self-criticism, and feelings of inadequacy. You can create a life full of self-love by listening to your inner voice and living your absolute best life!

Chapter 6

TINY STEPS FOR SUCCESS

Introduction

You learned how being in the present moment while eating can make a wonderful sensory experience out of your meal, and you explored the benefits of listening to your hunger and fullness cues. In this chapter, you will learn how to make these new practices and your changed thought patterns into wonderful new habits.

This chapter has three fundamental objectives:

- Show how tiny behaviors are the key to making long-lasting behavioral changes.
- Demonstrate how attaching these changes to anchor behaviors makes them easy to remember to perform.
- Explain how to celebrate your achievements and use those celebrations to reinforce your changes.

By the end of this chapter, you will know how to create lasting change that will help free you forever from Diet Culture. These changes will help you forge a new way of being—one that includes listening to yourself, being kind to yourself, and opening a world of food possibilities.

Section 1: What Are Tiny Behaviors?

Hazel is a professional woman with an accomplished career. The only area in which she did not feel accomplished was her weight. She never felt good enough or thin enough when she compared herself to her skinnier colleagues. Year after year, she found herself ensnared in the cycle of New Year's resolution dieting. The diets, always ambitious and stringent, were invariably given up by February. She was continually left feeling defeated and at a higher weight than when she started the diet.

Recognizing the need for change, Hazel reached out for my help. Hazel shared her struggles with me, her failed diets, the recurring weight gain, and the constant disappointment that accompanied those efforts.

I proposed a different approach. We talked about how drastic life and diet changes are usually doomed to fail. I showed her how making tiny, sustainable changes over time leads to healthier habits and better long-term weight management.

In the previous chapter, we explored the concept of mindfulness and mindful eating and recognized the importance of listening to the body. By adopting these practices, we can learn to eat when we are hungry, stop when we are satisfied, and enjoy whatever food we desire, whenever we wish.

Now, we will delve into the next fascinating topic: creating lasting behavioral changes, but with a twist. We are going to start small—tiny, even. We often fall into the trap of the all-or-nothing mindset when it comes to changing our eating habits. We decide to make drastic changes like "I will cut out all carbs" with the expectation that we will lose weight quickly and become super happy and admired by all.

But here is the hard truth: Maintaining such radical changes is usually not sustainable. For instance, when you attempt to eradicate carbs from your diet, you often end up feeling lethargic, foggy-brained, and irritable. It is a tough battle against cravings. You might give in, grabbing that bag of chips, promising to stop after just a few. But one thing leads to another, and before you know it, you have devoured the whole bag. Why is that?

The answer is simple: You set yourself up for failure.

Enormous behavioral changes tend to fail because they are simply too drastic, too unrealistic, and too difficult to sustain. Think back to past New Year's resolutions like "I am going to lose thirty pounds, quit smoking, run a marathon, and climb Mount Everest!" Like Hazel's goals, these goals lack specific and clear pathways to success. Instead of repeating those unsuccessful patterns, this time you are going to systematically build your success on a solid foundation.

> Enormous behavioral changes tend to fail because they are simply too drastic, too unrealistic, and too difficult to sustain.

In chapter 4, you learned to change your long-standing negative thoughts about yourself and food. You scrutinized those thoughts, created healthier replacements, and converted them into empowering mantras. Those mantras about yourself and your food signify new behaviors. In chapter 5, you discovered the science and joy of mindfulness and mindful eating. You practiced grounding yourself in your senses and learned a new way of eating with our mindful eating exercise. These new behaviors are a significant improvement over restrictive eating patterns that lead to binging. Now you need to take the next steps:

- Permanently incorporate your self mantras.
- Permanently adopt your food mantras.
- Make mindful eating a permanent habit.

The big question is, how do you ensure these behaviors stick?

You are going to make these changes systematically and give them clarity and purpose. You will begin by breaking the new habits into small, manageable steps. You will connect these habits to existing habits and allow them to grow organically. For example, proposing to recite your mantra out loud all day, every day, would be a massive undertaking and would be quite a hefty expectation to place on yourself. But you can create a more realistic goal for yourself, such as "I aim to practice my mantra for two minutes each day." That goal is far more achievable and thus more likely to become a consistent behavior.

You can apply the same logic to your new food mantra, "Carbs are healthy," which we crafted in chapter 4. Repeating this mantra constantly throughout the day is not feasible, but dedicating just one minute per day to this practice is much more manageable.

The same concept applies to mindful eating. Is it realistic to expect every meal or snack to be a leisurely, mindful experience? Probably not! We are all busy with our daily lives, kids demand our attention, and we need to find time to shower! So, how can you embed mindful eating into your routine? By making it a "tiny" habit. But how exactly do you do that?

You do this by establishing a small mindfulness check-in with yourself each day. This goal is less daunting than trying to make every snack and meal a mindful one and is more achievable. This is the sustainable way to integrate mantras and mindfulness into your life, and you can gradually amplify this behavior until it becomes second nature.

The beauty of tiny habits is that they are easy to implement daily.[1] Once something becomes easy, it is much simpler to solidify it as a habit and then add to it as you see fit. When you are feeling tired or stressed, it is often tempting to slip back into old, unhelpful behaviors and thought patterns. When your new behaviors are easy and small, it is simpler to get back on the right track if you momentarily deviate. That is the secret to creating lasting change. Hazel learned that she needed to incorporate small dietary changes and affirmative mantras to be able to create lasting, sustainable change. You can learn this too!

Remember: To instill long-lasting new behaviors, start with the smallest, simplest, and most achievable baseline behavior, something that you can easily perform. You can always scale it up later.

In the next section, we will delve into how to attach these new tiny behaviors to existing habitual behaviors. This approach will give you a consistent, built-in reminder to practice your new behavior, making the process of adopting new habits even more seamless.

Section 2: Creating Tiny Behaviors

Hazel started by focusing on one small change each week. The first week, Hazel committed to replacing her morning doom scroll on smart devices with two minutes of her mantra, "I am beautiful as I am." The next week, she started incorporating a one-minute mantra, "No food is off limits," before she ate breakfast. The following week, Hazel began a mindful snack-eating exercise. Each change seemed insignificant on its own, but over time they added up, creating a snowball effect of positive habits.

Throughout the process, Hazel faced challenges and setbacks, but I was there every step of the way, providing guidance and reassurance. I reminded Hazel that progress is not always linear, and every step, no matter how small, was a victory in itself.

Hazel was successful because she paired her tiny behavioral changes with existing anchoring behaviors—actions she was already doing each day. Anchoring behaviors serve as easy reminders to engage in a new behavior. In this way, she was able to create sustainable and long-lasting change.

Anchoring Behaviors

What is an anchoring behavior? An **anchoring behavior** is an existing habit or activity that occurs regularly and can act as a trigger for your new behavior.[2]

Brushing your teeth is one example of a common behavior that could be used as an anchoring behavior. I recall standing in front of the bathroom mirror as a child, observing my older sister diligently cleaning her teeth. That is how I picked up the practice. Over time, even without my sister present—though perhaps with occasional reminders hollered from the living room by my parents—I continued to brush my teeth. I found the minty freshness so pleasing that I actually enjoy the polishing part at the dentist (though not the rest of the appointment!). This ritual has since become an ingrained habit I perform twice daily.

You likely have similar memories and routines. Perhaps you have built toothbrushing into specific moments in your day. For example, you might rise at 8 am and head straight to the bathroom to brush your teeth. Maybe you have a more extended morning ritual. Mine begins with waking up at 7 am and then drinking a glass of water and a cup of coffee. This is followed by a bathroom break, exercise, a shower, brushing my teeth, styling my hair, applying makeup, dressing, preparing breakfast, and then setting off for work. Any one of these actions could serve as an anchoring behavior.

Anchoring Behavior Exercises

The secret to embedding a new habit into your routine lies in integrating it with an existing behavior. By attaching your new habit to an already established routine, it becomes an effortless part of your daily life.[3] You can use one of the new mantras you developed in chapter 4 to practice. For this exercise, I will use "I trust my body." A manageable way to integrate this mantra into daily life is to say it out loud for two minutes, once each day.

What anchoring behavior could I tether this to? Looking at

my morning routine, it seems natural to associate this mantra with waking up, when I am nestled safely in bed. When I add this new habit to an existing anchoring behavior, my refreshed routine might look like this:

1. Wake up and repeat the mantra "I trust my body" for two minutes.
2. Drink water and coffee.
3. Visit the bathroom, exercise, shower, brush teeth, fix hair, apply makeup (if needed), and dress.
4. Prepare breakfast.
5. Eat breakfast with my family.
6. Head off to work.

Doesn't that sound more manageable? I mean, I am just lying in bed, all cozy and safe. I can easily spend two minutes repeating that mantra. And what a serene way to commence the day!

I can do the same exercise with the mantra "Carbs are healthy." Devoting just one minute each day to repeating this mantra is a good stepping-stone toward transforming this mantra into a mental habit. I find that a fitting moment to recite this mantra is while preparing breakfast, which usually contains a carb or two. Therefore, the act of toasting my bread makes a good anchoring behavior for this mantra. While I wait, I can repeat my mantra for one minute. Thus, my morning routine now becomes:

1. Wake up and repeat the mantra "I trust my body" for two minutes.
2. Drink water and coffee.
3. Visit the bathroom, exercise, shower, brush teeth, fix hair, apply makeup (if needed), and dress.

continued

> 4. Prepare breakfast *while repeating the mantra "Carbs are healthy" for one minute while the bread is toasting.*
> 5. Eat breakfast with my family.
> 6. Head off to work.
>
> Pretty simple and achievable!

Anchoring behaviors serve as reminders that reinforce your new habits, just like brushing your teeth became an automatic part of your routine long ago. This is a much healthier practice than fostering negative thoughts about yourself and those evil carbs.

What about your new mindful eating habit? You can effortlessly integrate this habit into any mealtime with a simple exercise. It does not have to be breakfast, but that might be an ideal time to shape your new dietary mindset.

Envision yourself sitting at a table, alone or with others, without any other distractions. Take a moment to breathe in and out slowly. Assess your level of hunger and your overall feelings. Admire the food before you, taking in its visual appeal and fragrance. Take a moment to express gratitude. Then take your first bite, savoring the taste and texture. Continue to enjoy your food until you start to feel satiated. Recheck your feelings and gauge your level of fullness.

Here is my new complete morning routine:

1. Wake up and repeat the mantra "I trust my body" for two minutes.

2. Drink water and coffee.
3. Visit the bathroom, exercise, shower, brush teeth, fix hair, makeup (if needed), and dress.
4. Prepare breakfast while repeating the mantra "Carbs are healthy" for one minute.
5. Eat breakfast *mindfully* with my family.
6. Head off to work.

How do you feel about this adjusted morning routine? Personally, I think incorporating these three behaviors into my morning routine is a breeze. After all, I am already eating, so why not eat mindfully instead of getting distracted by the TV or scrolling aimlessly on my phone? The act of reciting mantras and eating mindfully is so calming and revitalizing, it feels like I have already refreshed myself before my workday even begins. Hazel added these behaviors to her routines, and they helped her successfully change her eating behaviors.

Next, we will learn how to ensure these habits stick with us for a lifetime.

Section 3: Making It Stick!

How is Hazel doing now?
Over time, these small changes had a significant impact on Hazel. She noticed she was feeling more energetic and healthier. She also realized she had started losing weight, but this time it felt different. It was not the result of a punishing, restrictive diet, but the outcome of adopting healthier habits and a more positive relationship with food.

More importantly, Hazel began to appreciate her body, not for how it looked, but for all the incredible things it allowed her to do. She was kinder to herself and celebrated every tiny victory, every little change, without the pressure of meeting a drastic New Year's resolution.

Hazel's story serves as a reminder that big changes start small. A series of small steps can lead to significant transformations. Her story also demonstrates the importance of seeking professional help when stuck in harmful cycles. With patience, support, and guidance, Hazel was able to break free from the cycle of New Year's dieting resolutions and embrace a healthier, more sustainable lifestyle. And for the first time in many years, Hazel welcomed the new year not with a restrictive resolution but with a commitment to continue her journey of health and self-love.

In the previous section, you did an exercise that showed you how to embed small behavioral modifications into your daily routine. In this section, we will explore how the potent influence of reinforcement can make these habits stick for a lifetime.

To understand this concept, we need a brief history lesson about behaviorism and a notable figure named B. F. Skinner.

B. F. Skinner was a trailblazer who devoted his scientific work to comprehending human behavior, particularly how behavior is reinforced or curtailed through reward or punishment.[4] His findings indicated that both positive and negative reinforcement could increase the frequency of a behavior. Here, it is crucial to note that "positive" and "negative" do not denote "good" or "bad." Rather, *positive* implies adding or giving, while *negative* implies subtracting or taking away.

Positive reinforcement is like a reward. For instance, when you completed all your chores as a child, your mom may have praised you or given you some money. That is positive reinforcement. **Negative reinforcement**, on the other hand, can be thought of as relief or removal of an irritant. A common example is the cessation of the persistent reminder sound in your car when you fasten your seat belt.

Both types of reinforcement can motivate us to repeat those behaviors—one offers a delightful reward, the other provides relief from a minor annoyance. Studies indicate that positive reinforcement tends to be a more robust and long-lasting strategy for creating enduring habits.

You might also be familiar with Skinner's revelation that behaviors can decrease in frequency through both positive and negative punishment. **Positive punishment**, despite seeming contradictory, simply means the addition of a punitive consequence. For example, if you were impolite to your parents, they might have reprimanded you—that is positive punishment. **Negative punishment**, conversely, entails taking something away. If you threw a tantrum, your parents might have confiscated your toys or iPad or perhaps sent you to time-out. Positive punishment adds a punitive element, while negative punishment removes something cherished.

Interestingly, Skinner found that punishment was not an effective long-term strategy for eliminating a behavior. If the goal is to entirely **extinguish** a behavior, neither rewards nor punishments should be applied. Instead, the behavior should be ignored or extinguished. For instance, if a mother consistently disregards a child's tantrums, the child may initially increase the intensity of the tantrums, but eventually, if all tantrums are ignored, the behavior typically ceases.[5]

How can you apply these scientific principles to change your thoughts and ensure the changes become ingrained? First, you develop the capacity to redirect or eliminate your unwanted behaviors by consciously refraining from engaging in them. This involves altering your thought patterns and deliberately avoiding reverting to past thinking habits. An example of this might be ceasing to soothe yourself with a pint of ice cream when you are feeling down. These previous thought patterns and their resultant behaviors are gradually being eliminated. As a result, you no longer resort to punitive measures such as undergoing a physiologically dangerous five-day juice cleanse to pay for your ice cream "sins."

In the process of making these changes, you shape new behaviors and transform them into habits. One effective way to solidify these new behaviors is to consistently reward yourself each time you successfully execute them. You might imagine the need to offer yourself a substantial reward each time you adhere to the new behavior. But, as with major behavioral transformations, substantial rewards might not be practical. Instead, smaller rewards or forms of celebration are often more realistic and equally effective.[6]

What does a mini celebration entail? It could be any action or affirmation that helps you acknowledge the significance of the moment while providing you with a dose of positive reinforcement. In doing so, you enhance the likelihood that the behavior will become habitual.

> ### Making-It-Stick Exercise
>
> How do you make your new habits stick? Through the application of behavioral science principles and the technique of positive reinforcement! To illustrate, think back to the previous exercise in which you started using the mantra "I trust my body." The anchor behavior was waking up. Before getting out of bed, you recite your "I trust my body" mantra for two minutes. Right after you finish, you are going to celebrate! You can do any of the following actions or come up with your own:
>
> - You can simply say, "Well done!" or "Great job!"
> - You can give yourself a hug.
> - You can remind yourself of your awesomeness.
> - You can assume a confident pose as you prepare your morning coffee.

Find a method of celebration that resonates with you. The act of celebration serves to positively reinforce your new behavior and transform it into a routinely performed habit.

Why does this work? It works because the positive feelings you experience after completing a task encourage you to repeat that action more frequently. You can use these minor celebrations to solidify new behaviors and make them into habits by regularly providing positive reinforcement. You are not restricted to one form of celebration. You should feel free to vary your celebrations daily, but ensure that they are meaningful and affirming.

Remember these concepts:

- Significant behavioral changes are challenging to sustain because they require considerable effort and are difficult to implement.
- Simplifying the new behaviors, trimming them down into tiny steps, and associating them with existing habits makes them manageable and achievable.
- Treating yourself to a small celebration or reward helps you reinforce these behaviors through the power of positive reinforcement.

These concepts can be represented as a simple equation:

> Anchoring Behavior + New Behavior + Celebration = Permanent New Habit!

This combination of behavior creates a framework for creating enduring change. Even if you only manage to perform the minimum requirements of your new behaviors, you have a reason and an opportunity to celebrate. What if you accomplish more? Then, you should celebrate even more! There is no limit on what you can add to this process. I recommend starting with the minimum because even if you only achieve your basic goals, you still always have a reason to celebrate. Any additional accomplishments are simply a bonus. Therefore, each day becomes a celebration, even when you are just practicing your smallest new habits. These are the lessons that Hazel learned, and now she is on her way to loving herself as she is and celebrating all her small successes.

In our final chapter, we will consolidate all this knowledge, explore how we can build on these newfound successes, and discuss how to recover if you regress or fail to maintain your new habits. You will be well on your way to rendering Diet Culture obsolete while cultivating a healthier, more compassionate mindset that celebrates success.

Chapter 7

ADDING ON AND PREVENTING RELAPSE

Introduction

I hope you found chapter 6 to be an invaluable resource that will help you create tiny behaviors that can latch onto anchors and make them last a lifetime by celebrating your successes.

You should congratulate yourself for reaching the final chapter. We'll wrap up with a brief review and outline helpful and positive ways to prevent a **relapse** (falling back into old behaviors and habits after a behavioral change occurred) into Diet Culture. We have three fundamental objectives:

- Review the lessons presented by looking at Liam's journey.
- Learn how to add on to your tiny behaviors to increase your new positive habits.
- Find compassionate and helpful ways to prevent relapse.

By the end of this chapter, you will be forging your way to a happier and healthier way of thinking, feeling, and behaving. You will have regained your appreciation and love of all foods and will have learned how to eat mindfully. You will be on your way to making lasting habits that are positive and healthy. You will have successfully reprogrammed yourself into a new and healthy relationship with food and a healed mind, and you will be well on your way to living a diet-free life for good!

Section 1: Adding On!

For the final stage of our journey together, let me share an inspiring story about Liam.

Life had thrown many curveballs at Liam, leaving him with unhealed emotional scars, a struggle with body image, and a tumultuous relationship with food. Liam grew up in an emotionally abusive household with a father who berated him for his weight and called him horrible names. This caused Liam to find solace and comfort in food, which only exacerbated the issues between him and his father. He learned early that he would only receive love from his father if he was thin. This set him on an emotionally difficult path toward dieting and overexercising. He tried countless diets and exercise regimens only to find himself bouncing back to his old habits, each failure reinforcing his negative self-image. Dejected but determined to change his life for the better, he mustered the courage to take a significant step toward healing and came to see me.

First, we looked at the science of why diets don't work so that he could see that he was not the failure, the diets were. (We covered these topics in chapter 1.) I helped him see that his body is his staunch ally, fiercely fighting against extreme weight-loss strategies. We talked about how Lookism and Weightism biases manipulate our perceptions, embedding the false notions that thin equals good and fat equals bad. We cleared away the fog surrounding Diet Culture and its perpetual cycle of self-doubt and criticism. In addition, I had Liam detox his social media feeds, stop watching advertisements, and limit time within toxic relationships. First and foremost, he had to learn how to create healthy boundaries with his father. He began gravitating slowly toward body positivity and self-compassion.

Then we started to work on creating a new relationship with food. (We covered these topics in chapter 2.) Liam looked to his past to understand his eating habits as a child and his difficult relationship with his father. We identified where he was eating emotionally and mindlessly, and learned how to differentiate between those behaviors and true physical hunger. Liam also learned to stop labeling foods as bad or good and to simply see food as food, which set him on a path toward a healthier relationship with food.

I helped Liam reconnect with his body's signals of hunger and satiety, and he learned what happens when we neglect these cues. (We covered these topics in chapter 3.) We practiced differentiating true hunger from emotional or mindless eating. We gained insights into the roles of ghrelin and leptin, our hunger and satiety hormones. Finally, Liam learned that overeating, restricting, or eating when not hungry could lead to cravings and addictive food behaviors.

I introduced Liam to the concept of Cognitive Behavioral Therapy (CBT) and explained how our thoughts, feelings, and actions are intricately connected and influence each other. (We covered these topics in chapter 4.) Over the course of several sessions, Liam learned how his distorted beliefs about himself and food had paved the way for his unhealthy eating habits. I guided him through the process of identifying and challenging these deep-seated beliefs and replacing them with healthier, more rational ones. This was not easy for Liam, as his father's name-calling and abuse had etched deep scars within his heart.

As difficult as it was for Liam, I had him engage in positive self-talk and introduce helpful and healing mantras into his routine. And we reinforced these new patterns of thinking by having him place handy sticky note reminders of these mantras around his space.

Mindfulness was a game-changer for Liam. It taught him to savor his food, pay attention to his body's needs, and notice the emotional triggers that led him to overeat. He started practicing mindful eating with just one meal a day, finding the experience surprisingly enjoyable and gratifying. This tiny act of mindfulness began to ripple through his daily habits, influencing his choices and behaviors. (We covered these topics in chapter 5.)

I then introduced Liam to the concept of tiny behavioral changes, explaining how small, sustainable changes could lead to significant transformation over time. We identified achievable goals that aligned with Liam's new, healthier mindset. He learned to anchor these new behaviors to his existing daily routines by creating a schedule for mantra recitation and his mindful eating practice. We explored the joy of celebrating these achievements, using positive reinforcement to cement these behaviors into habits. (We covered these topics in chapter 6.)

Over time, Liam started to see himself and his relationship with food in a whole new light. He was no longer trapped in the cycle of failed diets and self-criticism. He had found a new path—one of self-love, mindfulness, and healthy habits. His journey was not without bumps and hurdles, but the tools and strategies he had learned equipped him to navigate those hurdles with resilience.

So, what if you, like Liam, now want to take your healing process a step further? By now, you likely have a few mantras that you are comfortably repeating after your habitual activities, and you are probably incorporating mindful eating into your daily routine. I am sure it feels wonderful to see your happiness meter rising as you consistently and easily perform these new habits. Are you ready for more?

Here is the key: Keep the changes tiny. Sometimes our enthusiasm can lead us to set ambitious goals, which may leave us feeling deflated when they prove too challenging to stick to. Think about Hazel's New Year's resolution scenario, where grand promises sound appealing but are often hard to keep. You are already in the process of transforming deeply ingrained negative thoughts about yourself and food. Don't lose your focus on the changes you have made that are leading you to success. Instead, think about what else in your life could benefit from a makeover. Perhaps you have found yourself saying some of these things:

- "I want to find more time for exercise."
- "I want to eat healthier foods."
- "I want to stop obsessively checking my body in the mirror."

These are all fantastic goals! But they are a bit broad, are they not? We need to break down these objectives into tiny, achievable behaviors that we can seamlessly integrate into our lives.

We'll start with the goal Liam wanted to add, which is a

common one: "I want to find more time for exercise." (Please keep in mind that before you start any exercise regimen, you should consult your doctor to find the right forms that work for you.)

I have been a Pilates fitness instructor since 2003, and I can attest that finding a regular exercise routine can do wonders, not only for your physical health, but your mental health as well. But many people will create this as a vague goal ("I want to find more time to exercise.") They will find sporadic times to try to achieve their goal, but they will then find it too hard to do regularly. They then slack off and fail to achieve their goals.

The way to avoid this outcome, like we learned in chapter 6, is to make this behavioral change TINY!

How much exercise could feasibly become part of your daily routine? Think about this and keep the goal realistic—consider the busyness of your life, the amount of free time you have, the best time of day for you to exercise, and the daily activity that could serve as your anchor for this new behavior. This is what I had Liam explore.

Liam expressed a desire to focus on cardio, as he felt that running helped him release extra tension and work through negative emotions. He always felt less burdened and more clearheaded after a good run. But he always struggled with finding the time to fit a run into his busy schedule.

What is the ideal amount of time to exercise? Most doctors would recommend adding about thirty minutes of exercise to your day. This feels achievable to many, but Liam felt he had less time available. Because he felt exceptionally busy, he set a goal of twenty minutes and found this to be much more suitable. He remembered that when adding a new behavior, it was best to start small with a duration that he knew he could commit to every day, or at least three to four days per week.

Next, he had to determine what habit could serve as his anchor for this behavior. He decided that doing this first thing after waking up and drinking water was best. He tried it out and used his watch to track his exercise, which conveniently celebrated his achievement after the twenty-minute mark. Upon trying this, he found that running for twenty minutes was doable and easy, and he found ways to celebrate his success by making himself a delicious breakfast after his run and toasting himself with his favorite creamy latte.

Since adopting this routine, he found that there were only a couple of days when he could not follow through, typically due to travel or other significant commitments. It became his exercise baseline, and he found that any additional time spent running was a delightful bonus.

I encourage you to take some time to identify a couple of new goals that you can transform into tiny behaviors. This simple technique prevents stagnation and promotes consistency, ensuring these new behaviors are manageable and sustainable. When you see these small changes becoming permanent, effortless habits, you will be filled with a sense of accomplishment and joy. This might be a feeling you have not encountered for a while.

We have been swamped by Diet Culture's promises of quick solutions, instant fixes, magic pills, and injections to make our weight and image concerns disappear. But when you learn how to gradually transform old, unhealthy habits and mindsets into healthier, simpler, and sustainable new habits, you will find even more reasons to leave Diet Culture behind. At this point, you possess all the tools necessary to do exactly that. You should be extremely proud of the strides you are making on this journey toward a healthier, more self-compassionate life.

> When you learn how to gradually transform old, unhealthy habits and mindsets into healthier, simpler, and new sustainable habits, you will find even more reasons to leave Diet Culture behind.

Before we wrap up, let us address a crucial topic: relapse prevention. It is important to know how to navigate any instances where you might find yourself sliding back into Diet Culture and forgetting to practice self-love.

Section 2: Preventing Relapse

Liam realized he had been a captive of Diet Culture for many years. And, although he considered himself healed, he understood he was also susceptible to relapse. When faced with the desire to "body check" himself critically in front of a mirror or consider the latest breakthrough diet medication, he realized that relapse was only a moment away. To prevent this, he incorporated three powerful practices into his life: grounding, meditation, and self-compassion.

He began with grounding. A simple yet potent practice, **grounding** involves reconnecting with the physical world around us, typically through the senses. Liam started small, using his morning wake-up routine to incorporate a mini grounding exercise.

Next, he explored meditation. Initially, the idea was a little daunting, but he started with just five minutes a day. Gradually, he increased the duration as his comfort with meditation grew. Over time, Liam noticed that his recurring thoughts of dieting became less overwhelming. He was learning to acknowledge them without letting them control his actions.

Last, Liam turned his attention to self-compassion. This was perhaps the most challenging part of his journey. After years of internalizing Diet Culture's often harsh rhetoric, he had to relearn how to speak to himself with kindness. He made a point of counteracting every negative thought with a positive affirmation. Whenever he caught himself falling back into old patterns, he would remind himself "I am human, and it is okay to stumble. What matters is that I am making progress."

Causes of Relapse

Maintaining rigorous standards can lead to feelings of failure and disappointment, which is the same defeatist mentality that Diet Culture often induces. You need to equip yourself with the tools needed to rebound if (or when!) you veer back toward Diet Culture. Remember, it is normal to stumble, but with self-love and kindness, these hiccups will not define your journey.

At the outset of any lifestyle change, momentum is high, largely fueled by novelty and enthusiasm. But as with many New Year's resolutions, when we make sweeping promises without a realistic, long-term plan, we tend to revert to old patterns. Escaping Diet Culture is a significant behavioral shift because it involves shedding ingrained negative thinking, dieting habits, food misconceptions, and self-deprecating attitudes. This type of transformation requires patience and persistence.

You have already established manageable and sustainable new habits, like repeating new mantras at consistent times and practicing mindful eating. These new behaviors are crucial because they are now the default mechanisms that you can rely on if any new habit you have tried to incorporate starts to falter.

But why would you relapse? Various triggers could cause a relapse: an envy-inducing bikini photo posted by a high school adversary on Instagram, a news article about the latest miracle weight-loss medication that convinces you that medication is the solution to your weight concerns, or a tactless comment from a gossip-loving colleague that sends you spiraling toward comfort food.

Life is unpredictable, and you never know what might nudge you back into old patterns. That is where your new baseline habits come in handy. In moments of stress, despair, or when you find yourself teetering on the edge of Diet Culture, you can lean on these small but meaningful behaviors. Celebrating each completion will help you regain your balance.

Think of these tiny habits as your safety net. They act as grounding mechanisms, helping you return to your center and stay the course. But what if you are triggered and need more? Some people feel regular therapy is beneficial and find that it helps them actively work on these triggers and explore viable solutions. But if therapy is not readily available to you, the following exercises may help in such moments to keep you from sliding back into Diet Culture. They helped Liam, and I know they can help you too!

Meditation

In addition to the mindfulness exercises in this book on page 89, there are fantastic resources such as the Calm and Headspace apps that offer a respite from the whirlwind of daily life while helping you cultivate a meditation practice.

Meditation, a calming and centering activity that allows you to slow down your mind and provides relief from anxiety and depression, has been instrumental in my personal journey. During graduate school, I turned to meditation as a way to manage the stress and anxiety I faced. I realized I needed to connect with my breath and body in a way that not only offered immediate relief but also provided a long-term strategy for stress management. I encourage you to discover your own unique path to meditation.

There is no one-size-fits-all approach when it comes to meditation. Some styles may feel too restrictive or challenging to sustain. See what resonates with you. Personally, I found solace in a soothing piece of music and prefer to meditate lying down. But remember, meditation can be done while walking, sitting, or even standing. You might choose to repeat mantras, focus on cultivating loving-kindness, or concentrate on your breath.

Regardless of the method you choose, the benefits of meditation are plentiful. Here are a few of the profound benefits I have experienced:

- Enhanced multitasking capabilities
- Heightened empathy and compassion
- Improved stress management
- Better overall physical and mental health
- Increased emotional intelligence

Remember, a regular meditation practice can be rejuvenating, bring calm and peace, and help you align more deeply with your body and mind. You will become more aware of what you need in the moment. There will be times when triggers might cause you to revert to old maladaptive patterns, automatically lean into negativity, or bring up unpleasant memories. These are the moments when you might be particularly hard on yourself, spiraling into self-destructive behaviors. During those times, turn to meditation for assistance. It can help you avert the negative spiral and help avert a relapse. Liam found this helped him, and he particularly resonated with the following exercise.

> ### Meditative Body Scan Exercise
>
> Either read from the exercise below or visit our Meditations web page to participate in this exercise by pointing your phone's camera at the QR code below and following the link to our Meditation Videos page at anew-insight.com.
>
> This meditation is helpful to connect you to your physical body while releasing tension and stress.
>
> 1. Lie down in a comfortable place on your bed, couch, or floor. Adjust your body until you feel your muscles relaxing and releasing all tension and stress. Feel your body connected to what you are sitting on or lying upon while gently and slowly breathing in and out.
> 2. Bring greater awareness to your breath, and breathe slowly in and out. Breathe in, and breathe out.
> 3. Imagine for a moment that you are flying high above the clouds, floating effortlessly and weightlessly. Soar high, free, and unencumbered.
> 4. As you float high above the clouds, bring awareness to your feet. Move your awareness over your feet and toes, your arches, and the balls of your feet. Move up slowly through your ankles, up your shins, into your

calves. As your awareness travels up your body, feel each part that your awareness touches relax and release all tension in that area of your body.

5. Bring your awareness to your knees and thighs. Feel your thighs melt under your awareness as you move to your hips and buttocks. Let go of any tension and stress.

6. Rising higher up your body, find your awareness in your belly, and imagine your stomach muscles and your organs warm and relaxed.

7. Move higher up to your chest, relaxing your pectoral muscles and your shoulders. Let your awareness travel down your arms and your hands. Let go of the tension in your arm muscles down to each fingertip. Feel the warmth around your wrists, and let the stress spill out from your fingertips.

8. Moving up to your neck, allow the warmth and the relaxation to continue up to your jaw, your mouth, your cheeks, your eyes, your forehead, and the crown of your head.

9. Now bring your awareness to your entire body as you float high above the clouds. Feel how much lighter and freer you feel after releasing and relaxing your entire body. As you float high above the earth, allow yourself to relax further until you are free of stress, tension, and the worries of your day.

10. Bring your awareness back to your breath. Breathe slowly in and out. Breathe in; breathe out.

11. Let your mind come back to your room. Slowly allow yourself to open your eyes. Remember this feeling of floating effortlessly high above the clouds, relaxed, tension-free, without any stress or care in the world.

Self-Compassion

Another way to combat a relapse into Diet Culture is to practice **self-compassion**. As you can see from chapter 4, you have been conditioned to be your own worst enemy, berating and belittling yourself for not fitting into an impossible standard. Just like changing your thoughts to truer, healthier, and more positive thoughts, practicing self-compassion can be a necessary salve against the damaging messaging that comes from Diet Culture. If you can remind yourself that you are whole and a wonderful human being just as you are, you can continue to reject the messaging that comes from Diet Culture. Liam found the following exercise helped him greatly to reconnect to the loving part of himself.

Self-Compassion Exercise

The first step is to recognize when you are starting to spiral and fall back into self-destructive behaviors. When you notice this happening, this exercise will help you navigate back toward self-compassion. This exercise helped Liam return to a place of calm and peace, and I hope it can help you realign with self-love and kindness. Either read from the exercise below or visit our meditations web page to participate in this exercise by pointing your phone's camera at the QR code below and following the link to our Meditation Videos page at anew-insight.com.

1. Find a moment to sit comfortably in a chair.
2. Breathe in slowly and breathe out slowly.
3. Imagine you are outside of yourself, floating above your body for a moment.
4. Try to imagine you are seeing yourself for the first time.
5. Note what you are seeing: a beautiful person, struggling for a moment, sad or triggered, and needing to find self-compassion.
6. Now, silently repeat the following phrase three times to yourself as you float above your body:
    a. "May I have peace. May I have joy. May I have kindness. May I have love."
7. Focus now on your heart. Fill it with peace, joy, kindness, and love.

Know in your heart you deserve these things because you are a good, kind person, worthy of all these blessings. Try to perform this act of self-compassion on yourself every time you feel triggered, sad, lonely, or angry or whenever something has pulled you off your path of self-care. Remember, you are doing your absolute best in this life. You are a loving friend and family member. You are a person who deserves love, empathy, and compassion.

Throughout your life, you have been inundated by the messages of Diet Culture—you have been constantly told you are not good enough, thin enough, rich enough, happy enough, or deserving enough. You have spent almost your entire lifetime trying to live up to an unrealistic ideal that cannot make you happy. You know that this is a dead-end street. But now you are wiser, more enlightened, and filled with insight. You have forged a new path to reach your goals, found novel ways to be kind to yourself, discovered how to honor your body and mind, and learned how to be more present in the moment. All of these steps will help you on your journey toward happiness.

And you deserve to be here.

Liam's transformation took time, but he saw that these small and achievable steps paved the way to his healthier relationship with himself and his food. I hope you are making the same revelations as you deprogram yourself out of Diet Culture. As we conclude this part of the journey, you should feel proud of all you have learned and the changes you have initiated. Escaping the clutches of Diet Culture is an immense accomplishment, and here you are, doing it with grace and self-compassion.

Section 3: Closing Thoughts

Abigail's Happy Ending

Remember Abigail? I introduced you to her in the preface to this book. She was a picky eater as a child but was pressured by her parents to clean her plate at mealtimes. Abigail lost touch with her inherent ability to self-regulate and, after gaining weight in puberty and becoming a target for school bullies, Abigail decided dieting was the answer. By the time she was a teenager, she was fully immersed in Diet Culture which, of course, failed her time after time. This pattern continued into adulthood, which made her mentally and physically exhausted and caused her self-esteem to plummet. Eventually, she came to me looking for a better way.

Abigail began her therapy sessions with me learning about the scientific and psychological reasons why cycles of restrictive dieting do not work and eventually lead to weight gain. She also learned about the negative sociological and cultural factors that influence us in Diet Culture. Once Abigail saw that dieting was an effort in futility, she understood that it might not be the answer to her issues with her weight. We then examined her childhood relationship with herself and food and looked at how that influenced her current relationships. We also worked through the erroneous and harmful negative thoughts she had about herself and food, and we formulated new, healthier, and more productive thoughts for her to practice and incorporate instead. Abigail then learned how to better listen to her body by relearning her hunger and fullness cues, and she adopted a mindful eating practice. All these changes were incorporated using the latest, most effective strategies for behavioral change.

Abigail gained knowledge and power as she naturally started to lose weight. She was astonished that she could eat whatever she wanted, whenever she wanted, and still lose weight. She escaped Diet Culture, learned to trust herself, and found a freedom like she had never known before. And that is what I want for you, too.

Next Steps

I am so proud of you for embarking on this journey, and I feel confident you now have the skills to move forward on this path with ease and grace. But do not feel you have to do this alone. Recruit others!

Find like-minded people with whom you can share this knowledge. Encourage them to read this book and help themselves escape from the unhealthy mentality that has kept them trapped and unhappy. Take our online course Deprogram Diet Culture® and solidify the lessons learned in this book with helpful and informative videos, exercises, a beautiful photography-filled workbook, and more. Go to anew-insight.com and enter the code DDC15 for a $15 discount.

It is my hope that we will be beacons of light, illuminating the way for others to be kind to themselves and honor their body and mind and to realize the power within to make lasting changes in their lives. This is my hope for you, and I know you have the power to make this a lasting change for the better in your life.

Thank you for trusting me and allowing me to join you during this part of your new journey.

As always,
I wish for *you to be well.*
I wish you *peace.*
I wish you *joy.*
I wish you *kindness.*
I wish you *love.*

GLOSSARY

Adaptive Thermogenesis: A process that slows metabolism during weight loss and causes the body to resist the decrease of fat levels. (Chapter 1, Section 1)

Anchoring Behavior: An existing behavior or event that occurs at a regular interval that can serve as a reminder for you to perform your new behavior. (Chapter 6, Section 2)

Anorexia Nervosa: Behavior characterized by extreme self-starvation, having a fear of gaining weight, possessing an extremely low body weight, and experiencing body dysmorphia. (Chapter 2, Section 3)

Appearance Anxiety: Excessive worry about how you look. (Chapter 1, Section 3)

Attachment Theory: How the caregiver–child relationship emerges and influences mental, physical, and emotional development. (Chapter 2, Section 1)

Binge Eating Disorder: Behavior characterized by a negative self-evaluation, binge eating larger than normal amounts of food in a discrete (usually two-hour) time period, feeling a lack of control over one's eating, and feeling distress over the binges that occur at least one day per week for three months. (Chapter 2, Section 3)

Body Dysmorphia: A perception that certain parts of your body are larger than they actually are. (Chapter 1, Section 3)

Body Energy Partitioning System: An adaptive system that considers the ratio of fat to lean muscle tissue the individual person has in the beginning of the diet and determines, in equal proportions, the amount of fat or lean muscle lost during the diet. (Chapter 1, Section 1)

Body Positivity: An overarching love and respect for the body that allows individuals to

(a) appreciate the unique beauty of their body and the functions that it performs for them;

(b) accept and even admire their body, including those aspects that are inconsistent with idealized images;

(c) feel beautiful, comfortable, confident, and happy with their body, which is often reflected as an outer radiance, or a glow;

(d) emphasize their body's assets rather than dwell on their imperfections; and

(e) interpret incoming information in a body-protective manner whereby most positive information is internalized and most negative information is rejected or reframed. (Chapter 1, Section 3)

Bulimia Nervosa: Behavior characterized by a negative self-evaluation and binge eating larger than normal amounts of food. (Chapter 2, Section 3)

Clean Eating: Eating food free from pesticides, additives, preservatives, and impurities in a way that promotes cleansing and purifying the body. (Chapter 2, Section 3)

Cognitive Behavioral Therapy (CBT): A type of therapy focused on understanding how your thoughts affect your feelings, which subsequently dictate your behaviors. (Chapter 4, Section 1)

Cognitive Distortions: Misinterpretations or exaggerations of situations. (Chapter 4, Section 1)

Compensatory Hyperphagia: The amount we eat after deprivation. (Chapter 1, Section 1)

Diet Culture: A rigid set of expectations about valuing Lookism over physical health and emotional well-being and the motivations and actions behind the push to achieve that ideal form. (Chapter 1, Section 2)

Emotional Eating: When certain emotional states affect how and what we eat. (Chapter 2, Section 2)

Extinguish: Ignoring a behavior so it is eliminated completely. (Chapter 6, Section 3)

Ghrelin: A hormone made and released primarily from the stomach. It is known as a hunger-producing hormone. (Chapter 3, Section 3)

Grounding: A mechanism that helps reduce stress and return you to a calm place. (Chapter 5, Section 1)

Hunger: A metabolic state that is defined by the lack of nutrients or energy, characterized by a motivation and/or verbalization of the need to obtain food due to physiological signals from the body that indicate the need to eat. (Chapter 3, Section 1)

Hunger Signals: Stomach growls and pains, weakness, headache, dizziness, anxiety, grumpiness, difficulty concentrating, cravings, thirst, and a watering mouth. (Chapter 3, Section 1)

Leptin: A hormone released from the fat cells that helps us regulate our food intake over time. (Chapter 3, Section 3)

Lookism: A subtle form of prejudice based solely on physical appearance. It leads to preferential treatment of "better-looking people" over those considered not good looking. (Chapter 1, Section 2)

Maladaptive Schema: A long-standing, long-lasting, and dysfunctional or self-defeating pattern of thinking developed in childhood or adolescence that informs a negative belief about the self, the world, or the future. (Chapter 4, Section 1)

Mantras: A form of meditation that involves continually repeating a specific word or phrase while passively tuning out any other type of internal or external distraction. (Chapter 4, Section 3)

Meditation: A calming and centering activity that allows you to slow down your mind. It provides relief from anxiety and depression. (Chapter 7, Section 2)

Mindful Eating: A focused, open-hearted, and nonjudgmental awareness of food, free of any consideration of whether the food is good or bad for us. (Chapter 5, Section 2)

Mindfulness: Being aware of the present moment and accepting it in a nonjudgmental, open-hearted manner. (Chapter 5, Section 1)

Mindfulness-Based Cognitive Therapy (MBCT): A type of therapy that attempts to change depressive ruminative thinking about the past or anxiety regarding the future by switching from the "doing mind" to the "being mind." (Chapter 5, Section 1)

Mindfulness-Based Eating Awareness Training: A combination of self-regulation and increased mindfulness to address oversensitivity to emotional, social, or behaviorally conditioned cues, such as advertising and peer pressure. It helps us key in to the body's hunger and fullness signals. (Chapter 5, Section 2)

Mindless Eating: When we eat in a distracted environment without conscious awareness or attention to our food. (Chapter 2, Section 2)

Negative Affect: Sad and despondent facial expressions. (Chapter 1, Section 3)

Negative Perfectionism: The unhappy pursuit of the thin ideal. (Chapter 1, Section 3)

Negative Punishment: Having something taken away that has the effect of decreasing a behavior. (Chapter 6, Section 3)

Negative Reinforcement: An action viewed as a relief that has the effect of reinforcing a behavior. (Chapter 6, Section 3)

Orthorexia Nervosa: Obsessive preoccupation with healthy nutrition or reaching a certain body ideal to the point where it impairs a person's ability to have a positive social life or it impacts their health and nutrition. (Chapter 2, Section 3)

Positive Punishment: Adding a punishment that has the effect of decreasing a behavior. (Chapter 6, Section 3)

Positive Reinforcement: A reward that has the effect of reinforcing a behavior. (Chapter 6, Section 3)

Post-Starvation Fat Overshooting: A phenomenon directed by the sympathetic nervous system that considers body weight, food intake, and body composition as determinants of what weight will be regained over the body's original weight set point after significant weight loss. (Chapter 1, Section 1)

Relapse: Falling back onto old behaviors and habits after a behavioral change occurred. (Chapter 7, Introduction)

Repetitive Negative Thinking (Rumination): Obsessively thinking the same negative thought to the point of dysfunction and/or impairment. (Chapter 4, Section 1)

Satiation: Feeling satisfied on a physiological level. No longer hungry but not stuffed. The desire to eat and its associated hunger signals cease, and food appears to lose its attraction. (Chapter 3, Section 1)

Self-compassion: Extending compassion to oneself in instances of perceived inadequacy, failure, or general suffering. (Chapter 7, Section 2)

Self-regulation: Paying attention to internal physical and emotional cues. (Chapter 3, Section 1)

Suppressed Thermogenesis: The body's process during periods of deprivation that adapts and slows down fat loss to increase the body's ability to survive. (Chapter 1, Section 1)

Sympathetic Nervous System: The body's fight-or-flight nervous system that increases heart rate, blood pressure, breathing rate, and pupil size. It also causes blood vessels to narrow and digestive juices to decrease. (Chapter 1, Section 1)

Thought Stopping: A technique from Cognitive Behavioral Therapy that is meant to help people stop their negative thoughts and adopt new, healthy thoughts. (Chapter 4, Section 3)

Weightism: Bias against people considered overweight or obese. (Chapter 1, Section 2)

NOTES

Chapter 1

1. Abdul G. Dulloo, Jean Jacquet, and Jean-Pierre Montani, "How Dieting Makes Some Fatter: From a Perspective of Human Body Composition Autoregulation," *Proceedings of the Nutrition Society* 71, no. 3 (August 2012): 379–89, https://doi.org/10.1017/S0029665112000225.

2. Dulloo, Jacquet, and Montani, "How Dieting Makes Some Fatter."

3. Dulloo, Jacquet, and Montani, "How Dieting Makes Some Fatter."

4. Dulloo, Jacquet, and Montani, "How Dieting Makes Some Fatter."

5. Chris Warhurst et al., "Lookism: The New Frontier of Employment Discrimination?," *Journal of Industrial Relations* 51, no. 1 (February 2009): 131–36, https://doi.org/10.1177/0022185608096808.

6. A. Janet Tomiyama, "Weight Stigma Is Stressful. A Review of Evidence for the Cyclic Obesity/Weight-Based Stigma Model," *Appetite* 82 (November 2014): 8–15, https://doi.org/10.1016/j.appet.2014.06.108.

7. Natasha A. Schvey, Rebecca M. Puhl, and Kelly D. Brownell, "The Impact of Weight Stigma on Caloric Consumption," *Obesity* 19, no. 10 (October 2011): 1957–62, https://doi.org/10.1038/oby.2011.204.

8. Danielle Couch et al., "Obese People's Perceptions of the Thin Ideal," *Social Science & Medicine* 148 (January 2016): 60–70, https://doi.org/10.1016/j.socscimed.2015.11.034.

9. Schvey, Puhl, and Brownell, "Impact of Weight."

10. Couch et al., "Obese People's Perceptions."

11. Schvey, Puhl, and Brownell, "Impact of Weight."

12. Tracy L. Tylka, "Overview of the Field of Positive Body Image," in *Body Positive: Understanding and Improving Body Image in Science and Practice*, ed. Charlotte H. Markey, Elizabeth A. Daniels, and Meghan M. Gillen (Cambridge: Cambridge University Press, 2018), 6–33, https://doi.org/10.1017/9781108297653.002.

13. Nichole L. Wood-Barcalow, Tracy L. Tylka, and Casey L. Augustus-Horvath, "'But I Like My Body': Positive Body Image Characteristics and a Holistic Model for Young-Adult Women," *Body Image* 7, no. 2 (March 2010): 106–16, https://doi.org/10.1016/j.bodyim.2010.01.001.

14. Rachel Cohen et al., "#bodypositivity: A Content Analysis of Body Positive Accounts on Instagram," *Body Image* 29 (June 2019): 47–57, https://doi.org/10.1016/j.bodyim.2019.02.007.

15. Ornella Corazza et al., "The Emergence of Exercise Addiction, Body Dysmorphic Disorder, and Other Image-Related Psychopathological Correlates in Fitness Settings: A Cross Sectional Study," ed. Rachel A. Annunziato, *PLOS ONE* 14, no. 4 (April 3, 2019): e0213060, https://doi.org/10.1371/journal.pone.0213060.

16. Lucy Macfarlane, Glynn Owens, and Borja del Pozo Cruz, "Identifying the Features of an Exercise Addiction: A Delphi Study," *Journal of Behavioral Addictions* 5, no. 3 (September 2016): 474–84, https://doi.org/10.1556/2006.5.2016.060.

Chapter 2

1. Jane Ogden et al., "Distraction, the Desire to Eat and Food Intake. Towards an Expanded Model of Mindless Eating," *Appetite* 62 (March 2013): 119–26, https://doi.org/10.1016/j.appet.2012.11.023.
2. Ogden et al., "Distraction."
3. Allan Geliebter and Angela Aversa, "Emotional Eating in Overweight, Normal Weight, and Underweight Individuals," *Eating Behaviors* 3, no. 4 (January 2003): 341–47, https://doi.org/10.1016/S1471-0153(02)00100-9.
4. Geliebter and Aversa, "Emotional Eating."
5. American Psychiatric Association, ed., *Diagnostic and Statistical Manual of Mental Disorders: DSM-5*, 5th ed. (Washington, DC: American Psychiatric Association, 2013).
6. Chelsea Cinquegrani and David H. K. Brown, "'Wellness' Lifts Us above the Food Chaos': A Narrative Exploration of the Experiences and Conceptualisations of Orthorexia Nervosa through Online Social Media Forums," *Qualitative Research in Sport, Exercise and Health* 10, no. 5 (October 20, 2018): 585–603, https://doi.org/10.1080/2159676X.2018.1464501.
7. Hellas Cena et al., "Definition and Diagnostic Criteria for Orthorexia Nervosa: A Narrative Review of the Literature," *Eating and Weight Disorders—Studies on Anorexia, Bulimia and Obesity* 24, no. 2 (April 2019): 209–46, https://doi.org/10.1007/s40519-018-0606-y.

Chapter 3

1. Shauna L. Shapiro and Gary E. Schwartz, "The Role of Intention in Self-Regulation," in *Handbook of Self-Regulation* (Elsevier, 2000), 253–73, https://doi.org/10.1016/B978-012109890-2/50037-8.

2. Richard D. Mattes and Mark I. Friedman, "Hunger," *Digestive Diseases* 11, no. 2 (1993): 65–77, https://doi.org/10.1159/000171402.

3. Mattes and Friedman, "Hunger."

4. Mattes and Friedman, "Hunger."

5. Catherine Gibbons et al., "Issues in Measuring and Interpreting Human Appetite (Satiety/Satiation) and Its Contribution to Obesity," *Current Obesity Reports* 8, no. 2 (June 2019): 77–87, https://doi.org/10.1007/s13679-019-00340-6.

6. V. Somogyi et al., "Endocrine Factors in the Hypothalamic Regulation of Food Intake in Females: A Review of the Physiological Roles and Interactions of Ghrelin, Leptin, Thyroid Hormones, Oestrogen and Insulin," *Nutrition Research Reviews* 24, no. 1 (June 2011): 132–54, https://doi.org/10.1017/S0954422411000035.

7. Ariana M. Chao et al., "Stress, Cortisol, and Other Appetite-Related Hormones: Prospective Prediction of 6-Month Changes in Food Cravings and Weight: Stress, Cravings, and Weight," *Obesity* 25, no. 4 (April 2017): 713–20, https://doi.org/10.1002/oby.21790.

8. Somogyi et al., "Endocrine Factors."

9. Somogyi et al., "Endocrine Factors."

10. Kirk Warren Brown and Richard M. Ryan, "The Benefits of Being Present: Mindfulness and Its Role in Psychological Well-Being," *Journal of Personality and Social Psychology* 84, no. 4 (2003): 822–48, https://doi.org/10.1037/0022-3514.84.4.822.

11. Christian H. Jordan et al., "Mindful Eating: Trait and State Mindfulness Predict Healthier Eating Behavior," *Personality and Individual Differences* 68 (October 2014): 107–11, https://doi.org/10.1016/j.paid.2014.04.013.

Chapter 4

1. Aaron T. Beck, "A 60-Year Evolution of Cognitive Theory and Therapy," *Perspectives on Psychological Science* 14, no. 1 (January 2019): 16–20, https://doi.org/10.1177/1745691618804187.

2. Beck, "A 60-Year Evolution."

3. Beck, "A 60-Year Evolution."

4. Jennifer S. Coelho, Anita Jansen, and Martine Bouvard, "Cognitive Distortions in Normal-Weight and Overweight Women: Susceptibility to Thought-Shape Fusion," *Cognitive Therapy and Research* 36, no. 4 (August 2012): 417–25, https://doi.org/10.1007/s10608-011-9372-0.

5. Margarita Sala, Leigh C. Brosof, and Cheri A. Levinson, "Repetitive Negative Thinking Predicts Eating Disorder Behaviors: A Pilot Ecological Momentary Assessment Study in a Treatment Seeking Eating Disorder Sample," *Behaviour Research and Therapy* 112 (January 2019): 12–17, https://doi.org/10.1016/j.brat.2018.11.005.

6. Beck, "A 60-Year Evolution."

7. Gary Maria Bakker, "In Defence of Thought Stopping," *Clinical Psychologist* 13, no. 2 (July 2009): 59–68, https://doi.org/10.1080/13284200902810452.
8. Julie Lynch et al., "Mantra Meditation for Mental Health in the General Population: A Systematic Review," *European Journal of Integrative Medicine* 23 (October 2018): 101–8, https://doi.org/10.1016/j.eujim.2018.09.010.
9. Lynch et al., "Mantra Meditation."

Chapter 5

1. Jon Kabat-Zinn, Leslie Lipworth, and Robert Burney, "The Clinical Use of Mindfulness Meditation for the Self-Regulation of Chronic Pain," *Journal of Behavioral Medicine* 8, no. 2 (June 1985): 163–90, https://doi.org/10.1007/BF00845519.
2. J. Kabat-Zinn and R. Burney, "The Clinical Use of Awareness Meditation in the Self-Regulation of Chronic Pain," *Pain* 11 (1981): S273, https://doi.org/10.1016/0304-3959(81)90541-8.
3. James O. Prochaska and John C. Norcross, *Systems of Psychotherapy: A Transtheoretical Analysis*, 8th ed. (Stamford, CT: Cengage Learning, 2014).
4. Jean L. Kristeller and C. Brendan Hallett, "An Exploratory Study of a Meditation-Based Intervention for Binge Eating Disorder," *Journal of Health Psychology* 4, no. 3 (May 1999): 357–63, https://doi.org/10.1177/135910539900400305.
5. Kristeller and Hallett, "An Exploratory Study."

6. Jean Kristeller, Ruth Q. Wolever, and Virgil Sheets, "Mindfulness-Based Eating Awareness Training (MB-EAT) for Binge Eating: A Randomized Clinical Trial," *Mindfulness* 5, no. 3 (2014): 282–97.

Chapter 6

1. B. J. Fogg, *Tiny Habits: The Small Changes That Change Everything* (Boston: Houghton Mifflin Harcourt, 2019).

2. Fogg, *Tiny Habits*.

3. Fogg, *Tiny Habits*.

4. B. F. Skinner, "The Evolution of Behavior," *Journal of the Experimental Analysis of Behavior* 41, no. 2 (March 1984): 217–21, https://doi.org/10.1901/jeab.1984.41-217.

5. Skinner, "The Evolution of Behavior."

6. Fogg, *Tiny Habits*.

INDEX

A

adaptive thermogenesis, 9, 141
advertising
    influence on eating habits, 32
    limiting consumption of, 16–17
all-or-nothing thinking, 72, 103–104
anchoring behaviors
    defined, 107, 141
    pairing tiny behaviors with, 107–110, 126
anorexia nervosa, 43, 141
appearance anxiety, 24, 141
attachment theory, 33, 141
Aversa, Angela, 38
awareness. *See also* mindful eating
    of eating habits, 36
    and mindfulness, 89
    of negative thoughts, 76–77, 82
    and self-regulation, 50–51
    tuning in to body through, 61–63

B

"bad" food, dropping label of, 41–43
beauty
    body positivity, 21–23, 142
    embracing different forms of, 19
    Lookism, 13, 14–15, 143
    Weightism, 13–15, 20–21, 146
Beck, Aaron T., 67, 68
behaviors. *See also* tiny behaviors
    anchoring, 107–110, 126, 141
    extinguishing, 114, 143
    reinforcement and punishment, effect on, 113–114
"being mind," 88–89
binge eating disorder
    defined, 43, 141
    as example of emotional eating, 37–38
    Mindfulness-Based Eating Awareness Training for, 92–93
    and relationship with food, 31, 35, 40
body, listening to. *See also* mindful eating
    overview, 46–48, 122
    relearning about hunger and fullness, 49–53
body dysmorphia, 20, 24, 43, 142
body energy partitioning system, 8–9, 142
body image, societal standards regarding, 11–15
body positivity, 21–22, 142
body scan exercise, 132–133
Bowlby, John, 33
bulimia nervosa, 43, 142

C

carbohydrates, changing negative thoughts related to, 75–76
CBT (Cognitive Behavioral Therapy), 67–68, 73, 87, 142
celebrations, for adherence to new behaviors, 114–117
celebrity exercise routines, 23–24
Cena, Hellas, 44
childhood relationship with food
    and hunger and fullness cues, 50
    influence on present relationship with food, 35
    overview, 31–34
clean eating, 40, 43–44, 142
Cognitive Behavioral Therapy (CBT), 67–68, 73, 87, 142
cognitive distortions, 68–69, 72, 143
comfort eating, 35, 37, 49, 55
commercials. *See* advertising
compensatory hyperphagia, 10, 143
Covey, Stephen R., xii
cravings, understanding, 58–63

D

daily routine, incorporating tiny behaviors into, 108–111
demonization of food. *See* vilification of food
deprivation diets. *See* Diet Culture/dieting
Deprogram Diet Culture online course, 3–4, 138
deprogramming Diet Culture
    limiting advertisement consumption, 16–17
    overview, 12, 121–122
    reasons for dieting, 12–15
    reducing contact with toxic people, 17–18
    social media cleanup, 16
    steps in, 15
Diet Culture/dieting
    dawn of, 14
    deprogramming, 12–18, 121–122
    Diet Culture, defined, 143
    diet hamster wheel, 6–7, 10–11
    escaping cycle of, 137–138
    example of issues with, xix–xx
    overview, 1–4, 5, 22–23
    and post-starvation fat overshooting, 7–11
    reasons for, 12–15
    reprogramming mind in relation to, 19–27
    trends vilifying foods in, 42–43, 45
    and unhealthy cravings, 58–63
    why diets do not work, 6–11
digestion, hormones involved in, 59–61
distortions, cognitive, 68–69, 72, 143
distracted eating, 37, 54–55. *See also* mindless eating
"doing mind," 87–88
drastic changes, difficulty of achieving, 103–104
drugs for weight loss, 24–25

E

eating. *See also* emotional eating; mindful eating; mindless eating; relationship with food
    changing thoughts affecting, 75–76
    during childhood, 31–34
    clean, 40, 43–44, 142
    comfort, 35, 37, 49, 55
    distracted, 37, 54–55
    hormones involved in, 59–61

learning to stop vilifying food, 40–46
present habits, examining, 35–39
eating disorders. *See also* binge eating disorder
anorexia nervosa, 43, 141
bulimia nervosa, 43, 142
orthorexia nervosa, 44–46, 145
professional help for, 45
relation to extreme diets, 43, 45
emotional cravings, understanding, 58–63
emotional eating
defined, 37, 143
example of, 35
exercise related to, 39, 56–57
overview, 36, 37–39
stopping, 54–57
emotions
negative, emotional eating related to, 38
positive, finding in exercise routine, 25–26
exercise
punishing regimens, avoiding, 23–27
tiny behaviors related to, 124–126
external influences on childhood eating habits, 32
extinguishing, 114, 143

F

family, influence on eating habits, 32–34
fat overshooting, post-starvation, 7–11
fat shaming, 13–15
food, relationship with
changing thoughts affecting, 75–76
in childhood, 31–34

learning to stop vilifying food, 40–46
overview, 29–30, 122
in present, examining, 35–39
food cravings, understanding, 58–63
food industry, influence on eating habits, 32
fullness
exercise related to, 56–57
hormone involved in, 60–61
overview, 122
relearning about, 49–53

G

Geliebter, Allan, 38
ghrelin, 59–60, 143
goals, transforming into tiny behaviors, 124–126
"good" food, dropping label of, 41–43
grounding, 89–91, 128, 143

H

habits. *See also* tiny behaviors
creating, 105–106
making stick, 112–117
pairing with anchoring behaviors, 107–110
practice, role in forming, 82–83
Hallett, C. Brendan, 92–93
health. *See* reprogramming mind to improve health
hormones involved in eating and digestion, 59–61
hunger
defined, 143
exercise related to, 56–57
hormone involved in, 59–60
overview, 122
relearning about, 49–53

hunger signals, 51–52, 143
hyperphagia, compensatory, 10, 143

I
internal influences on childhood eating habits, 32–34
intuitive approach to eating. *See* mindful eating

K
Kabat-Zinn, Jon, 87
Kristeller, Jean, 92–93

L
leptin, 60–61, 143
listening to body. *See also* mindful eating
    overview, 46–48, 122
    relearning about hunger and fullness, 49–53
Long, Weldon, xi–xiii
Lookism, 13, 14–15, 143

M
making-it-stick exercise, 115
maladaptive schemas, 68, 144
mantras
    defined, 144
    pairing with anchoring behaviors, 107–110
    and role of practice in forming habits, 80–83
    tiny behaviors to permanently adopt, 105–106
MBCT (Mindfulness-Based Cognitive Therapy), 87, 92, 144

medications for weight loss, 24–25
meditation
    body scan exercise, 132–133
    defined, 144
    mantra, 80–81
    mindfulness grounding exercise, 89–91
    in relapse prevention, 128, 130–133
    self-compassion exercise, 134–135
mindful eating
    in childhood, 31–32, 34, 53
    defined, 92–95, 144
    overview, 46–48, 85, 122, 123
    pairing with anchoring behaviors, 110–111
    practicing, 96–99
    relearning about hunger and fullness, 49–53
    stopping emotional and mindless eating, 54–57
    tiny behaviors to permanently adopt, 105–106
    understanding unhealthy cravings, 58–63
mindfulness, 86–91, 144
Mindfulness-Based Cognitive Therapy (MBCT), 87, 92, 144
Mindfulness-Based Eating Awareness Training, 92–93, 144
mindless eating
    defined, 36, 144
    exercise related to, 39, 56–57
    versus mindful eating, 94
    overview, 36–37
    stopping, 54–57
mindset. *See* thoughts
morning routine, incorporating tiny behaviors into, 108–111

N

negative affect, 144
negative emotions, emotional eating related to, 35
negative perfectionism, 20, 145
negative punishment, 113–114, 145
negative reinforcement, 113, 145
negative thoughts
  changing, 72–77
  identifying, 66–71
  Thought Stopping, 79–80, 82
neutral mindset toward food, need for, 41–43
nutrient-dense foods, 62–63

O

Ogden, Jane, 37
online course, 3–4, 138
orthorexia nervosa, 44–46, 145
overweight persons, emotional eating by, 38
Ozempic, 24–25

P

perfectionism, negative, 20, 145
personalized mantras, 81
Pilates, 26
pleasure, finding in exercise routine, 25–26
positive content, repopulating social media feed with, 20–21
positive emotions, finding in exercise routine, 25–26
positive people, surrounding yourself with, 18
positive punishment, 113–114, 145
positive reinforcement, 113, 115–117

positive thoughts
  changing negative thoughts to, 72–77
  role of practice in shifting to, 78–84
Post-it notes, remembering mantras with, 83
post-starvation fat overshooting, 7–11, 145
practice, role in improving thoughts, 78–84
present relationship with food, examining, 35–39
punishing exercise regimens, avoiding, 23–27
punishment, and decrease in behaviors, 113–114

R

radical changes, difficulty of achieving, 103–104
reinforcement, role in making new habits stick, 112–117
relapse
  causes of, 129–130
  defined, 119, 145
  grounding in prevention of, 128
  meditation in prevention of, 128, 130–133
  overview, 128
  self-compassion in prevention of, 128, 134–136
relationship with food
  changing thoughts affecting, 75–76
  in childhood, 31–34
  learning to stop vilifying food, 40–46
  overview, 29–30, 122
  in present, examining, 35–39
repetitive negative thinking (rumination), 69, 145

reprogramming mind to improve health. *See also* thoughts
   body positivity, 21–22
   overview, 19–20, 22–23, 119–120
   punishing exercise regimens, avoiding, 23–27
   repopulating social media feed, 20–21
restorative exercise, 26
rewards for adherence to new behaviors, 114–117
rumination (repetitive negative thinking), 69, 145

S

satiation, 52–53, 122, 145
schemas, maladaptive, 68, 144
Schvey, Natasha A., 20–21
Schwartz, Gary, 50
self-compassion, 128, 134–136, 146
self-regulation, 50–51, 61–62, 93, 146
self-worth, improving sense of, 74–75
Shapiro, Shauna, 50
Skinner, B. F., 113–114
small behaviors. *See* tiny behaviors
social media
   cleaning up feed, 16
   repopulating feed with positive content, 20–21
societal standards regarding body image, 11–15
starvation, body's reaction to, 8–11, 51–52
stress reduction
   through exercise, 26
   through mindfulness, 87
supportive people, surrounding yourself with, 18
suppressed thermogenesis, 9, 146
sympathetic nervous system, 8–9, 146

T

thermogenesis
   adaptive, 9, 141
   suppressed, 9, 146
Thought Stopping, 79–80, 82, 146
thoughts. *See also* reprogramming mind to improve health
   making changes stick, 114
   negative and unhelpful, identifying, 66–71
   overview, 63, 65, 122–123
   positive, shifting to, 72–77
   practice, role in improving, 78–84
   role in eating, xi–xiii
tiny behaviors
   adding on to, 119, 121–127
   creating, 107–111
   defining, 103–106
   making new habits stick, 112–117
   overview, 101–102
   pairing with anchoring behaviors, 107–110, 126
   as safety net, 130
Tovar, Supatra, xi–xii, 1–4
toxic people, reducing contact with, 17–18, 83–84

U

underweight persons, emotional eating by, 38
unhealthy cravings, understanding, 58–63
unhelpful thoughts. *See* negative thoughts

V

vilification of food
    changing negative thoughts related to, 75–76
    clean eating, 43–44
    "good" and "bad" food labels, 41–43
    orthorexia nervosa, 44–46
    overview, 40

W

Wegovy, 24–25
weight gain after dieting, 7–11
Weightism, 13–15, 20–21, 146
weight-loss medications, 24–25
worthlessness, changing thoughts of, 74–75

Y

yoga, 26

THANK YOU FOR READING MY BOOK!

I really appreciate all your feedback, and I love hearing what you have to say.

I need your input to make the next version of this book and my future books better.

Please leave me a helpful review on Amazon letting me know what you thought of the book.

Thank you!

Dr. Supatra Tovar

Receive Our Free Resources!

Just to say thanks for buying my book, I would like to offer you digital copies of our *Deprogram Diet Culture Course Workbook*, our *Mindfulness Cookbook for Busy People*, AND our *Mindful Eating Journal* 100% FREE! These books are the first in a line of helpful tools under the ANEW Insight series focused on psychology, nutrition, and exercise and are helpful companions to *Deprogram Diet Culture: Rethink Your Relationship to Food, Heal Your Mind, and Live a Diet-Free Life*.

To receive your free digital copy of the *Deprogram Diet Culture Course Workbook*, please email us at connect@anew-insight.com and provide your invoice receipt for *Deprogram Diet Culture: Rethink Your Relationship to Food, Heal Your Mind, and Live a Diet-Free Life*, and we will email you a link to download our beautiful photography-filled course workbook absolutely FREE!

To receive your free digital copies of the cookbook and journal, go to the link below and enter your email address: https://anew-insight.com/free-ebooks/ and you will receive links to download these beautiful ebooks.

We hope you enjoy these resources and find them useful on your journey to deprogram out of Diet Culture. Here's to living a diet-free life forever!

Mindfulness Cookbook for BUSY PEOPLE

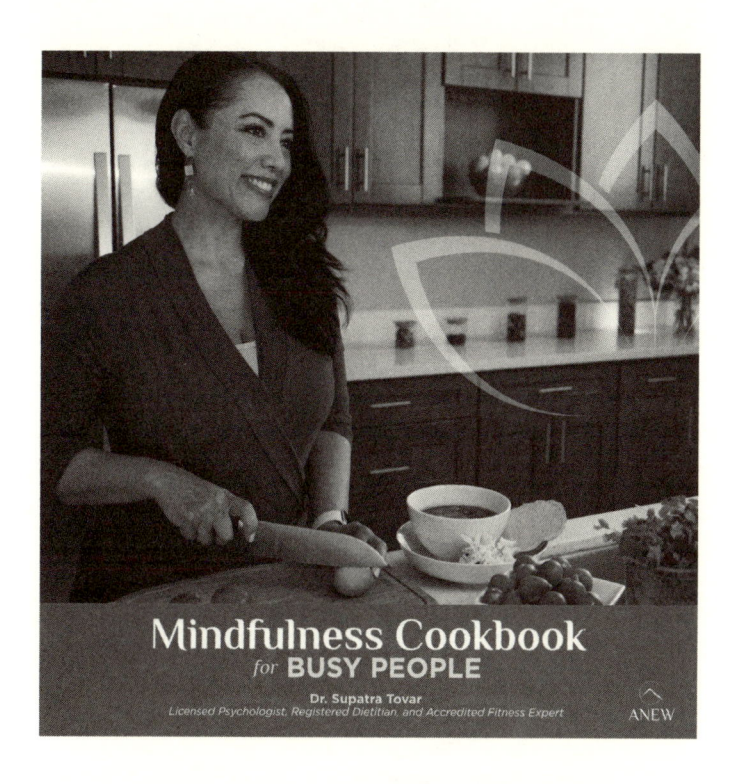

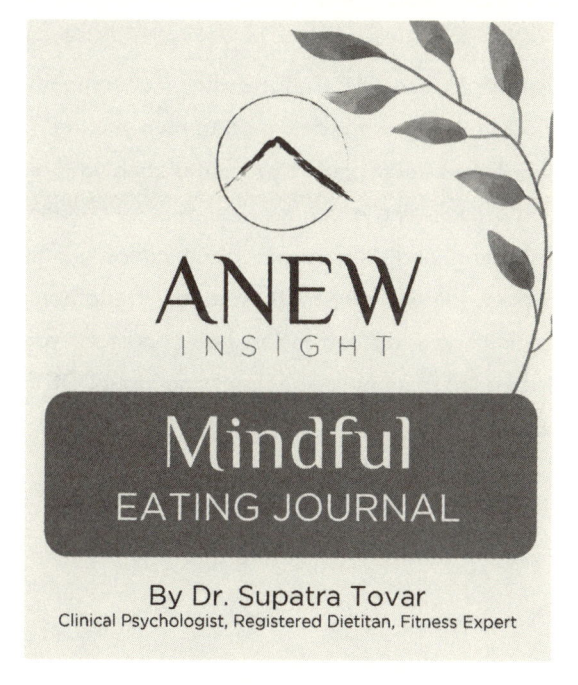

Dr. Supatra Tovar
Licensed Psychologist, Registered Dietitan, and Accredited Fitness Expert

ANEW

ANEW INSIGHT

Mindful EATING JOURNAL

By Dr. Supatra Tovar
Clinical Psychologist, Registered Dietitan, Fitness Expert

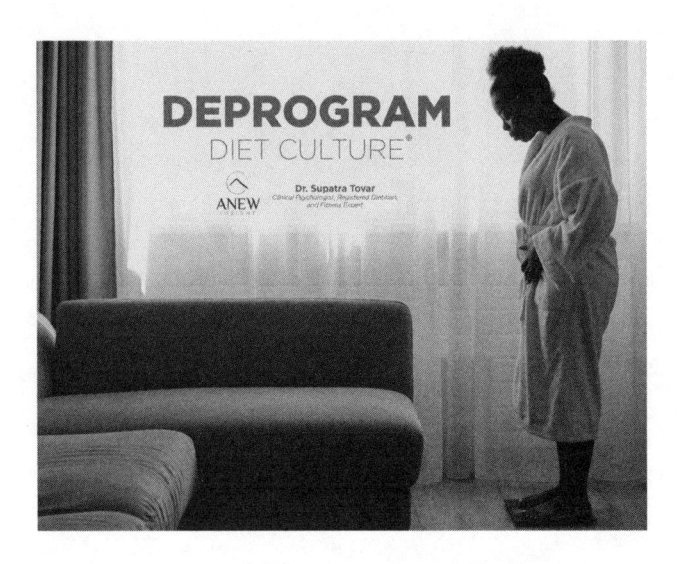

Take Our Online Course

Dr. Tovar converted her landmark program for a path to healing your relationship with yourself and food into a seven-step online video course, called Deprogram Diet Culture, with an accompanying workbook. This flagship program is designed to help you end frustrating cycles of dieting and weight gain by reformulating your relationship with food and establishing a stronger mind-body connection. With insightful, engaging, and thought-provoking videos, a digital and/or physical course workbook, and more, you can strengthen and reaffirm the principles you learned in this book and take your healing one step further. Go to anew-insight.com and input DDC15 for a $15 discount today!

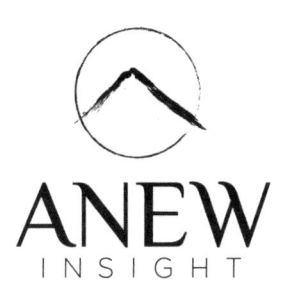

Follow Us!

Follow ANEW on social media:
Instagram: @my.anew.insight
TikTok: @my.anew.insight
YouTube.com/@my.anew.insight
Facebook.com/my.anew.insight
Threads: @my.anew.insight

ABOUT THE AUTHOR

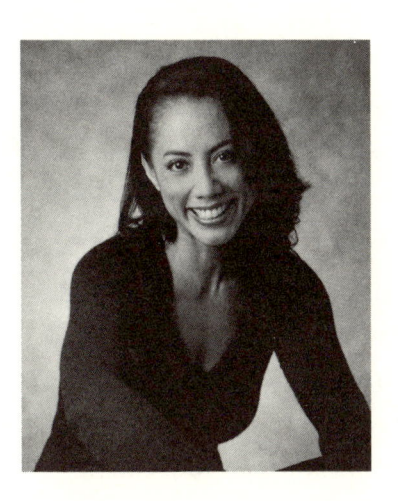

DR. SUPATRA TOVAR (PSY31949) is one of the only clinical psychologists who is also a registered dietitian and accredited fitness expert. Using research-proven techniques, Dr. Tovar has helped numerous clients overcome eating disorders, trauma, depression, and anxiety by teaching practical techniques that work for both the body and the mind. Her clients' successes led her to start ANEW, a company dedicated to guiding people through the journey of improving their relationships with the mind, body, and spirit.

Dr. Tovar has made numerous scholarly and professional presentations at several national conferences on a variety of health topics, including the detection and treatment of disordered eating, dissociation, weightism, health disparities among minorities, and mindfulness interventions for eating disorders.

Dr. Tovar has been interviewed by the most respected newspapers in the world, including the *Times* of London, the *Washington Post*, and the *New York Times*.

Dr. Tovar earned her doctorate in psychology from the California School of Professional Psychology and focused her postdoctoral training on the effects of trauma on health and disordered eating. Dr. Tovar also has a master of science degree in nutrition and a master of arts degree in psychology. She is a member of the Academy of Nutrition and Dietetics and the American Psychological Association, and has co-chaired the disaster response committee for the Los Angeles County Psychological Association. She opened her first private Pilates practice more than twenty years ago and has been a registered dietitian since 2015. For more information or to contact Dr. Tovar, please visit drsupatratovar.com.